NUTRITIONAL FACTORS IN GENERAL MEDICINE

Nutritional Factors In General Medicine
Effects of Stress and Distorted Diets

By

MARK D. ALTSCHULE, M.D.

Visiting Professor of Medicine, Harvard Medical School
Lecturer in Medicine, Yale University
Lecturer in Medicine, Boston University School of Medicine
President, Boston Medical Library
Biomedical Consultant, Office of Naval Research, Boston

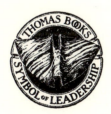

CHARLES C THOMAS · PUBLISHER
Springfield · Illinois · U.S.A.

Published and Distributed Throughout the World by
CHARLES C THOMAS • PUBLISHER

Bannerstone House
301-327 East Lawrence Avenue, Springfield, Illinois, U.S.A.

© *1978, by* CHARLES C THOMAS • PUBLISHER
ISBN 0-398-03736-1
Library of Congress Catalog Card Number: 77-13933

With THOMAS BOOKS *careful attention is given to all details of
manufacturing and design. It is the Publisher's desire to present books
that are satisfactory as to their physical qualities and artistic possibilities
and appropriate for their particular use.* THOMAS BOOKS *will be true
to those laws of quality that assure a good name and good will.*

Printed in the United States of America
W-2

Library of Congress Cataloging in Publication Data

Altschule, Mark David.
    Nutritional factors in general medicine.

    Includes bibliographical references and index.
    1.   Nutritionally induced diseases.   2.   Diet therapy.
3.   Nutrition.   I.   Title.   [DNLM: 1.   Nutrition.
2.   Stress.   3.   Diet—Adverse effects.   QU145 A469n]
RC622.A47   613.2   77-13933
ISBN 0-398-03736-1

This work is dedicated to
Eleanor Naylor Dana
whose moral and material support
led to its being written

INTRODUCTION

T HIS BOOK GREW out of four decades of clinical practice. This experience was in a measure given meaning and direction by the publications of many other clinicians. The book was written, however, because colleagues and students requested it after being made to appreciate concepts and interpretations that were at variance with some advanced by some professional nutritionists. The work will, therefore, consist of material observable by practitioners and useful to them.

Some readers may be surprised or disappointed to find some matters absent from this book. For example, there will be no general statements about the present status and future developments of clinical nutrition; these will be found in the papers by Peters,[1] Williams et al.,[2] Schneider and Hesla,[3] and Butterworth.[4] More specifically, the discussions will be limited largely to *nutritional* factors rather than to *dietary* factors. Hence, formal discussions of the treatment of gastrointestinal disorders will not be found here. Similarly, no formal discussions will be made of the biochemical disorders of severe kidney and liver diseases. All of these can be covered satisfactorily only in special treatises. Another subject that requires coverage in a special treatise is the increased vitamin needs in certain inborn errors of metabolism. Medical practitioners will rarely, if ever, see any of them, but they should, of course, know about them. The subject is well covered in the excellent review by Scriver.[5]

Another topic omitted from this book is the effects of food additives. The information available on this potentially alarming topic is not only too extensive and confused for concise discussion, but it is changing almost daily. Moreover, the subject is not specifically nutritional in nature and, hence, does not belong here.

The reader will find little in the way of biochemical discussion in this book. A serious—all but fatal—defect of the science of nutrition has been supersaturation with respect to subcellular biochemistry. If one shakes this mixture slightly, a cloud of processes consisting of electron transfers, coupled or uncoupled phosphorylation, mitochondrial and endoplasmic reticulum membrane changes—and of course DNA and RNA synthesis—all crystallize out. Since physicians rarely, if ever, are required to deal with any entity smaller than a patient, the biochemical discussions that make up much of the nutritional literature merely serve to distract and at times divert. Like the aurora borealis, they are impressive—even awe-inspiring—but not yet harnessed for use and, in any case, certain to vanish after a short existence. Accordingly, this material has been largely omitted here, only a small portion of it having been included in order to entice younger physicians into reading this book by providing them with something that sounds familiar. On the other hand, omitting all but small fragments of this vast literature has had beneficient effects: It has given us a thin book, one that can be comprehended by practicing physicians.

The exclusions listed above simplify the presentation of ideas considerably. There remain, however, two matters that require brief general discussion preliminary to the content of this clinical work. One deals with the effects of food processing. This has been discussed in two recent reports,[6, 7] but not very satisfactorily. One report[7] surprisingly states that "on an overall basis, the food preservation techniques in greatest use today do not result in major losses in the nutritive value of foods." This is quite different from what is found in the AMA monograph on the subject,[8] which cites an 80 percent loss in vitamins and minerals in the milling of grains and cereals. The Food Technologists' report[7] actually describes loss of vitamins A, B_1, C, and E during heat processing and drying. It also points out that processing plus pre-serving cooking (the latter is usually the more destructive) will remove a large part of the water-soluble vitamins such as thiamine, riboflavin, niacin, and ascorbic acid, so that only 35 to 45 percent remains. Surely these losses must be greater among those who cook carelessly at home (throwing away the cooking water) or eat in restaurants frequently. These matters are covered in the appropriate sections of this book. At any rate, these published data require modification of the statement that the American diet is the best in the world: It probably is when it is harvested, picked, or slaughtered, but any feeling of satisfaction owing to this fact must be submerged in what we know to be the results of processing and premeal cooking, which leave our diet outstandingly rich only in calories.

Another serious problem that practitioners must deal with is that created by the publication by official agencies of recommended daily allowances for the various nutrients. Actually, the problem of how physicians are to deal with the stated recommended daily allowances is easily solved. Since they are defined as the amounts adequate for "almost all healthy people," doctors need pay little attention to them, for doctors have little to do with healthy people. The words *almost all* have been defined as 97.5 percent of healthy people, a definition made manifestly absurd by the minute amount of data that has led to the formulation of the recommendations. The marked variability of even healthy people—a fact known at least to clinicians—makes it evident that authoritative recommendations can be valid only if made on very large numbers of people, which has not been done. Physicians, as they always have, will do the best they can for their patients unless prevented by administrative or judicial obtundity. The matter of when is a vitamin a food, a food substance, or a drug is discussed with some cynicism by Norman.[9] He points out that when a vitamin is present as less than 50 percent of the recommended daily allowance, it is called a food; if between 50 and 150 percent, a food supplement; and above that, a drug. By this definition, when 15 or 20 liters of water are given in a day to a patient with severe diabetic acidosis, it is a drug! Or when a patient with severe hyperthyroidism is given 200 percent of the normal caloric intake, all his food becomes a drug! A clinician is likely to consider such administrative definitions as useless in practice and insulting to the intelligence. Rather, he would prefer to hold that nutrients of any sort, when given in whatever amounts are required to ameliorate or prevent nutritional deficiency, can never be anything but nutrients. On the other hand, when the purpose is different, and a food substance is given so as to produce an effect that is not nutritional, it is best regarded as a pharmacologic agent, as is the case when vitamin D is given for hypoparathyroidism, or vitamin E for ischemic myositis (see page 154). Similarly under some circumstances, a common nutrient might become a poison, as is the case with meat, cheese, or milk in severe liver disease. In short, the nutritional treatment of patients is a proper duty of medical practitioners, and medical practitioners should determine what nutrients their patients need. The aim of this book is to present information that physicians can use in treating their patients.

REFERENCES

1. Peters, R. A.: The neglect of nutrition and its perils. *Am J Clin Nutr,* *26*:750, 1973.
2. Williams, R. J., Heffley, J. D., Yew, M.-L., and Bode, C. W.: A renaissance of nutritional science is imminent. *Perspect Biol Med, 17*:2, 1973.
3. Schneider, H. A. and Hesla, J. T.: The way it is. *Nutr Rev, 31*:233, 1973.
4. Butterworth, C. E., Jr.: The dimensions of clinical nutrition. *Am J Clin Nutr, 28*:943, 1975.
5. Scriver, C. R.: Vitamin-responsive inborn errors of metabolism. *Metabolism, 22*:1319, 1973.
6. Subcommittee on Food Technology of the Food Protection Committee, National Academy of Sciences: The use of chemicals in food production, processing, storage and distribution. *Nutr Rev, 31*:191, 1973.
7. Institute of Food Technologists Expert Panel on Food Safety and Nutrition and the Committee of Public Information: The effects of food processing on nutritional values. *Nutr Rev, 33*:123, 1975.
8. American Medical Association. *Nutrients in Processed Foods. Vitamins, Minerals.* Acton, Mass., Publishing Sciences Group, 1974.
9. Norman, C.: Vitamins, safety and freedom of choice. *Nature, 1*:244, 1973.

CONTENTS

PART V
MISCELLANEOUS TOPICS

NUTRITIONAL FACTORS IN GENERAL MEDICINE

PART I

ORGANIC MACRONUTRIENTS

CALORIES, OBESITY, WEIGHT REDUCTION, AND STARVATION

THE PROBLEMS OF human nutrition fall into two categories: (1) How much should a person eat? (2) What kind of food should one eat? A priori we should expect the answer to the first question to be clear and definite, whereas the answer to the second might be expected to be vague, uncertain, and fragmentary. In fact, the situation is just the reverse. As the later pages of this work will show, we know a great deal about specific nutritional needs. However, we have very little information on which to base an answer to the first question. The essential ambiguity of our understanding of how much we ought to eat was brought out in a recent article by Durwin of Glasgow and Edholm, Miller, and Waterlow of London.[1] Among other things, they pointed out that current assumptions that 70 percent of the world is undernourished in terms of calorie intake may be based on ignorance. The truth may be that in fact, 30 percent of the world—the 30 percent considered the standard—habitually eats too much, and that only a proportion, an unascertainable proportion, of the rest are actually undernourished. It is evident that some people can do very well on calorie intakes much less than officially recommended. Others may gain weight on such a regimen. Moreover, some persons can be given very large amounts of food with no increase in body weight. Contrarily, it is evident that some obese persons eat much less food than some who are lean and still do not lose weight. These contradictions defy explanation by currently available concepts.

A number of authors have discussed the roles of environmental and of genetic factors. It is well known that fat parents have fat children—but they also have fat pets. The brief but weighty discussion by Garn et al.[2] appropriately emphasizes the environmental factor—at least in a population in Michigan. However, fat babies do not necessarily grow up fat.[3] On the other hand,

5

taking the mammalia as a whole, there is no doubt about the importance of inheritance. A recent paper by James and Trayburn[4] reviewed the evidence of decreased heat production after eating and on exposure to cold. James and Trayburn[4] suggest that there is a genetically determined variation in glucose metabolism in skeletal muscles which leads to this deficiency in heat production, thereby leading in turn to obesity when food is available. (This genetic difference favors survival when food is scarce. Accordingly, after a period of famine, many of the survivors should become obese on refeeding, as is known to happen.) Although it is too soon to accept James and Trayburn's involvement of the specific enzyme system they suggest, the concept is nevertheless a good one. The finding of decreased calorigenesis in the obese continues to be corroborated.[5] A question, however, arises: Is the enzymic disorder necessarily inborn?

Attempts have been made to calculate human calorie requirements from energy expenditure. The assumption underlying this approach is that a normal, fully grown person, not pregnant, needs enough calories in the form of food and drink to provide the energy required by his or her way of life. However, the data show that for persons pursuing similar activities, the caloric requirement needed if weight is to remain unchanged may vary by as much as 100 percent. Moreover, as Edholm[6] has emphasized, it is useless to expect to be able to balance calorie intake as food against energy expenditure as work and heat production over the short term. On the other hand, when the figures for seven days of study are made into an average, calorie intake and energy expenditure are found to be close to each other. Nevertheless, the mechanisms whereby calorie intake and energy expenditure balance each other—as they do most of the time—are not understood. For example, the authors of a recent work,[7] psychologists, reviewed the endocrine aspects of the problem and, rejecting all previous theories, formulated their own which, however, will convince few endocrinologists. It is best at this moment to leave to one side the mechanisms of food-energy balance and pass directly to a consideration of the effects of overeating that produce weight gain.

To start with, it is necessary to emphasize that overeating is not a simple or even absolute matter. There is an important time factor. The number of meals into which the total calorie intake is divided is highly important—the fewer the meals, the greater the likelihood of obesity above minimal levels of intake. The patient who has essentially nothing for breakfast and little more for lunch but makes sure to take a large meal with meat, vegetables, and dessert in the evening is an excellent candidate for obesity despite what seems not to be an excessive calorie intake. In addition to these broad considerations there are many others, difficult to define, that suggest themselves. For each nutrient, the time of ingestion, the rates of digestion, of movement through the gut and of absorption must be taken into account. Sassoon[8] has analyzed these problems largely in terms of the enzymes involved. Whatever the validity of this analysis may or may not be, it does point to the complexity and subtlety of the problem. The factors discussed by Sassoon[8] offer a partial explanation for the impossibility of describing accurately the balance between food intake and energy production.

In addition, the effects produced by variations in physical activity, of the efficiency of muscle work, and of the amounts of muscle tension while resting must be considered, but they cannot for lack of data.

The effects of overeating are not easy to study, because when obese persons come in for observation, they are at a late stage of their metabolic disorder. In fact, by the time obesity has become established, many patients have ceased to overeat. Attempts have been made to study the metabolic consequences in non-obese persons of overeating for periods of one to three weeks;[9, 10] however valuable they may be in some respects, they are too short to contribute definitive data bearing on obesity. The best study of experimental overfeeding for our purposes is that reported by Sims et al.,[11] in which weight gain was induced over a six-month period. During the study, some of the subjects doubled their adipose tissue mass, and in some all of the weight gain showed up in the calculated fat mass. Exertional dyspnea developed with the obesity. Lassitude and decreased efficiency set in. The subjects fell into two groups: one consisted of persons who did not gain weight rapidly and who later lost it rapidly; the other group showed the reverse pattern. There was no explanation for this difference. Adipose tissue biopsy specimens were studied, and it was found in both groups that the fat cells increased in size and not in number. The serum cholesterol levels rose slightly, but not to abnormal levels. The serum triglyceride concentrations also rose, but exercise lowered them. Serum electrophoresis patterns did not change. A considerable rise in serum insulin level was found, despite which glucose tolerance was impaired, as shown by an excessive rise in serum insulin level after glucose feeding. The serum growth hormone response to glucose was, on the other hand, decreased. Cortisol secretion rates remained normal for size, although the serum levels fell slightly. The only difference from the pattern of spontaneous obesity seen in this experimental study was a decrease in plasma free fatty acid level. Once overeating became established, the metabolic pattern changed so as to favor fat deposition. The difficulty of securing weight reduction under these circumstances is evident. Generally similar results were found in a study of Japanese sumo wrestlers. Their strenuous regimen of physical activity is accompanied by a rigid dietary regimen. Unlike the normal Japanese diet of around 2300 calories in three meals, the sumo intake is 5000 calories in two meals.[12]

It must, however, be borne in mind that the hyperinsulinemia and the excessive rise in plasma insulin level are not inherent in obesity per se. When obese persons are fed high calorie diets low in carbohydrate, their insulin secretion falls toward normal.[13] After losing weight, the abnormal glucose metabolism of the obese returns to normal.[13, 14] However, this improvement is due only in part to the weight reduction and in part also to the low carbohydrate diet used during weight loss. Available evidence indicates that obese persons generate less heat than normal after glucose. The obese seemed to oxidize fat preferentially.[15] A program of diet modification combined with exercise, while it causes weight loss, need not change the serum lipid picture.[16]

One of the most distressing occurrences during attempts at weight reduction is that the loss slows with time. A decrease in energy expenditure occurs during the reducing regimen.[17] The mechanism appears to lie in the area of thyroid gland function.

During starvation, the circulating levels of triiodothyronine fall by 25 to 55 percent. The serum thyroxine levels show only insignificant decreases and the thyrotropic hormone none at all.[18] There seems to be an impairment of the ability of the body to change thyroxine to the hormone that acts at the cellular level, triiodothyronine. How to circumvent this mechanism is not immediately apparent.

Also confusing are changes in salt metabolism during fasting and refeeding. Fasting causes an immediate increase in urinary sodium excretion,[19] which is maximal on the fourth day and gone by the eighth. This phenomenon parallels the changes in serum glucagon level that accompany fasting, and glucagon is known to cause renal sodium loss. On the other hand, it must be borne in mind that although starvation causes increased aldosterone secretion, there is an accompanying lessened sensitivity of the kidney to that hormone. This phenomenon is said to explain the early salt loss of starvation.[20] If the fasting subject should take a considerable amount of carbohydrate, the salt-retaining effect of glucose would come into play at a time when aldosterone secretion is still high, and this might cause the surprisingly large gains in weight that dieting obese persons exhibit when they go off the diet. The salt-retaining effect of glucose is of unknown mechanism; it does not operate through aldosterone.[20]

The unhappy consequences of obesity are more than merely cosmetic. Obesity not only causes cor pulmonale directly, but it aggravates hypertension, coronary atherosclerosis, gallbladder disease, and the symptoms of arthritis. In addition, recent studies show that it may cause a severe nephrotic syndrome.[21] Accordingly, drastic attempts have been made to cure massive obesity using intestinal bypass operations. This procedure is often of only temporary benefit, and it may be responsible for decidedly harmful physiologic changes. It may cause temporary losses of potassium indicating wasting of muscle mass. The loss of muscle mass that may occur[22, 23] is accompanied by an increase in extracellular fluid volume, a finding typical of starvation. It causes severe liver disease, which may be fatal.[24, 25] One report states that this can be reversed by intravenous alimentation with amino acids,[26] but this awaits corroboration. Arthritis[27] and colonic pseudo-obstruction[28] are also consequences of the operation. In addition, the serum gastrin level rises and gastric acid secretion increases, despite which peptic ulcers do not seem to develop.[29] There is also a marked impairment of bile salt reabsorption, with resulting diarrhea and, more importantly, gallstone formation.[30] On the other hand, pulmonary function does improve.[31] The effects of the bypass operation are not merely to decrease absorption of food. Patients who have had the operation may exhibit decreased appetite.[32] (They also develop new food preferences.) Nevertheless, there is far from uniform satisfaction with jejunoileal bypass, and gastric bypass operations have been suggested.[33, 34] The operative treatment of obesity is not to be undertaken lightly.

What is to be done with the obese? Application of sociologic and psychologic techniques to study of the problem has revealed much of interest but little that is therapeutically useful.[35] Attempts to treat the disorder with low calorie diets should not work and, in fact, will not work at all in some cases even when adhered to.[36] Many obese persons cannot lose weight even with intakes of as little as 1000 calories daily. This discouraging fact makes it clear that no great progress can be made with the problem until the decrease in thyroid function that occurs with rigid dietary restriction can be circumvented. At present one hopeful approach seems to be total starvation under close supervision in a hospital, or else an evangelical approach analogous to alcoholics anonymous. Another approach that uses a diet of 400 to 800 calories per day plus strong "motivational enhancements" together with exercise is the Kempner regimen.[37] The food consists primarily of rice and fruit, so that over 90 percent of the calories come from carbohydrate. Vitamins are given. Since the sodium content of the diet is very low, the intake of water is restricted. On the other hand, the long-term results of behavioral therapy offer little cause for optimism.[38] Acupuncture, likewise, is ineffective,[39] as is the use of chorionic gonadotropin.[40]

It is evident that our understanding of obesity is fragmentary. Nevertheless, we must have at least temporary conceptual formulations. Garrow's masterly treatise[41] seems to offer what we need. Garrow starts with a distinction between homeostatic and buffering mechanisms. Homeostatic mechanisms operate minute by minute to maintain functions close to what is normal for that particular person. Blood chemistry values, body temperature, blood pressure, etc. are so regulated. When changes occur in either direction from the normal, mechanisms are quickly activated to counteract the force making the deviation and so prevent it. This does not apply to body weight. This measurement is not kept from changing minute by minute. Although fairly constant in the long run, it is highly variable day by day. Nevertheless, the tendency to vary is limited by a sort of buffering mechanism, which *resists* but does not *prevent* change. The more the deviation from the norm, the more the change is resisted, but the change is not totally prevented until an extreme is reached. Persons who lose weight by rigid dieting and who then cease their dieting subsequently regain weight to the same level, although they may overeat beyond that time. They can still attain a weight considerably above their normal, but they cannot go beyond a certain limit. Unfortunately, the nature of the buffering mechanisms remains to be defined.

Clinical experience teaches us that there are persons who gain weight easily and lose it with great difficulty. Are these the ones in whom a greater than average number of adipose cells are formed during intrauterine life? If so, we must regard obesity as a disease with a strong congenital, perhaps hereditary, predisposition. Above all, physicians should not fall into the trap of accepting the dogma, fashionable during the period 1930 to 1960, that in overeating, for every excess of nine calories, one gram of fat is inevitably laid down. This is certainly not inevitable and in fact rarely, if ever, happens.[42] This is because at least part of the excess calorie intake is dispersed as heat, a phenomenon that will not be detected if only the basal metabolic rate is measured.[43] Physicians who try to treat obesity should not make their task more difficult by calculating their anticipated results on the basis of irrational formulas.

Since the control of obesity is the regulation of the expression of appetite, it is possible that a way to regulate appetite may solve the problem. There is at present no certain way to do this over an extended period.*

---

* Physicians who want an account of the psychologic manifestations of obesity and of weight reduction by dieting or by intestinal bypass should read

RECOMMENDATIONS

Each adult should eat enough to reach or maintain the desired weight. If restriction of food is undertaken for long periods, highly processed foods (e.g. sugar as available in the market, processed starch foods) should be omitted and the intake of fat reduced.

STARVATION

Starvation owing to economic causes is rare in this country. When starvation occurs it is almost always a result of some recognizable disease, physical or mental. The wasting associated with certain metabolic or gastrointestinal diseases is easily understandable as the result of increased demand, decreased absorption, or impaired utilization of nutrients. Much less readily understood is the starvation associated solely with anorexia. Many diseases cause loss of appetite, but this is reversed with the onset of improvement. On the other hand, the mysterious extreme loss of appetite seen in patients with cancer or with psychiatric disorders defies comprehension. The severe anorexia of thiamine deficiency would also fall into this category if it were not for the fact that it is rapidly and completely reversed after the administration of the vitamin.

Whatever its mechanism, severe starvation produces a more or less standardized series of hormonal changes. The first is gonadal failure, manifested by amenorrhea in young women. Then follows thyroid failure. The marked fall in basal metabolic rate minimizes the weight loss and retards the development of vitamin deficiencies. A marked decrease in calorie intake causes a change in corticosteroid metabolism so that the urine 17-ketosteroid output falls, falsely suggesting adrenal failure. The adrenals do not fail.

When repletion occurs after starvation, the increase in metabolic activity may precipitate vitamin B and C deficiencies unless

Crisp, A. H., Kalucy, R. L., Pilkington, T. R. E., and Gazet, J. C.: Some psychosocial consequences of ileojejunal bypass surgery. *Am J Clin Nutr, 30*:109, 1977. Although there is little of practical value in it, the discussion is interesting in many ways, not the least of which is the fact that the word *unconscious* is not to be found in it.

added vitamins are given. During repletion there is a great need for additional nitrogen to restore lean tissue mass.

One aspect of starvation that has received little attention is its effect on serum bilirubin level. A marked reduction in calorie intake slows the excretion of bilirubin in both normal and jaundiced persons.[44] A disturbance in carbohydrate metabolism occurs in starvation and is discussed elsewhere (page 25).

REFERENCES

1. Durwin, J. V. G. A., Edholm, O. G., Miller, D. S., and Waterlow, J. C.: How much food does man require? *Nature, 242*:418, 1973.
2. Garn, S. M., Bailey, S. M., and Higgins, I. T. T.: Fatness similarities in adopted pairs. *Am J Clin Nutr, 29*:1067, 1976.
3. Poskitt, E. M. E. and Cole, T. J.: Do fat babies stay fat? *Br Med J, 1*:7, 1977.
4. James, W. P. T. and Trayburn, P.: An integrated view of the metabolic and genetic basis for obesity. *Lancet, 2*:770, 1976.
5. Kaplan, M. L. and Leveille, G. A.: Calorigenic responses in obese and non-obese women. *Am J Clin Nutr, 29*:1108, 1976.
6. Edholm, O. G.: Dietary data and estimates of energy expenditure. *Proc R Soc Med, 66*:641, 1973.
7. Woods, S. C., Decke, E., and Vasselli, J. R.: Metabolic hormones and regulation of body weight. *Psychol Rev, 81*:26, 1974.
8. Sassoon, H. F.: Time factors in obesity. *Am J Clin Nutr, 26*:776, 1973.
9. Nestel, P. J., Carroll, K. F., and Havenstein, N.: Plasma triglyceride responses to carbohydrates, fats, and caloric intake. *Metabolism, 19*:1, 1970.
10. Olefsky, J., Carpo, P. A., Ginsberg, H., and Reaven, G. M.: Metabolic effects of increased caloric intake in man. *Metabolism, 24*:495, 1975.
11. Sims, E. A. H., Goldman, R. F., Gluck, C. M., Horton, E. S., Kelleher, P. C., Rowe, D. W., and Elkinston, J. R.: Experimental obesity in man. *Trans Assoc Am Physicians, 81*:153, 1968.
12. Nishizawa, T., Akaoka, I., Nishida, Y., Kawaguchi, Y., Hayashi, E., and Yashimura, T.: Some factors related to obesity in the Japanese sumo wrestler. *Am J Clin Nutr, 29*:1174, 1976.
13. Grey, N. and Kipnis, D. M.: Effect of diet composition on the hyperinsulinemia of obesity. *N Engl J Med, 285*:827, 1971.
14. Jourdan, M., Goldbloom, D., Margen, S., and Bradfield, R. B.: Differential effects of diet composition and weight loss on glucose tolerance in obese women. *Am J Clin Nutr, 27*:1065, 1974.
15. Pillet, P., Chappins, P., Acheson, K., deTechtermann, F., and Jequiner,

E.: Thermic effects of glucose in obese subjects studied by direct and indirect calorimetry. *Br J Nutr, 35*:281, 1976.

16. Lewis, S., Haskell, W. L., Wood, P. D., Manoogian, N., Bailey, J. E., and Pereira, M.: Effects of plupical activity on weight reduction in obese middle-aged women. *Am J Clin Nutr, 29*:151, 1976.

17. Apfelbaum, M., Botsarron, J., and Lacatis, D.: Effect of calorie restriction and excessive calorie intake on energy expenditure. *Am J Clin Nutr, 24*:1405, 1971.

18. Merimee, T. J. and Fineberg, E. S.: Starvation-induced alterations of circulating thyroid hormone concentration in man. *Metabolism, 25*:79, 1976.

19. Boulter, P. R., Hoffman, R. S., and Arky, R. A.: Patterns of sodium excretion accompanying starvation. *Metabolism, 22*:675, 1973.

20. Kolanowski, J., Desmecht, P., and Crabbe, J.: Sodium balance and renal tubular sensitivity to aldosterone during total fast and carbohydrate refeeding in the obese. *Eur J Clin Invest, 6*:75, 1976.

21. Weisinger, J. R., Kempson, R. L., Eldridge, F. L., and Swenson, R. S.: Nephrotic syndrome: A complication of massive obesity. *Ann Intern Med, 81*:40, 1974.

22. Spanier, A. H., Kurtz, R. S., Shibata, H. S., MacLean, L. D., and Shizgal, H. W.: Alterations in body composition following intestinal bypass for morbid obesity. *Surgery, 80*:171, 1976.

23. Goldberger, J. H., Chung-Ja, Cha, Hazard, W. L., and Randall, H. T.: Jejunoileal bypass for morbid obesity: Early results and body composition changes in forty-five patients. *Surgery, 80*:493, 1976.

24. Mengla, J. C., Hoy, W., Kim, Y., and Chopek, M.: Cirrhosis and death after jejunoileal shunt for obesity. *Am J Dig Dis, 19*:759, 1974.

25. Holzbach, R. T., Wieland, R. G., Lieber, C. S., DeCarli, L. M., Koepke, K. R., and Green, G.: Hepatic lipid in morbid obesity. Assessment at and subsequent to jejunoileal bypass. *N Engl J Med, 290*:296, 1974.

26. Heimburger, S. L., Steiger, E., LoGerfo, P., Biehl, A. G., and Williams, M. J.: Reversal of severe fatty infiltration after intestinal bypass for morbid obesity by calorie-free amino acid infusion. *Am J Surg, 129*:229, 1975.

27. Wands, J. R., LaMont, J. T., Mann, E., and Isselbacher, K. J.: Arthritis associated with intestinal-bypass procedure for morbid obesity. *N Engl J Med, 294*:121, 1976.

28. Barry, R. E., Benfield, J. R., Nicell, P., and Bray, G. A.: Caloric pseudo-obstruction; a new complication of jejunoileal bypass. *Gut, 16*:903, 1975.

29. Solhaug, J. H. and Schrumpf, E.: Effect of small bowel bypass on serum gastrin levels and gastric acid secretion in man. *Scand J Gastroenterol, 11*:329, 1976.

30. Stein, T. A. and Wise, L.: Bile salt metabolism following jejunoileal bypass for morbid obesity. *Ann Surg, 185:*67, 1977.
31. Soterakis, J., Glennon, J. A., Ishibara, A. M., Tyler, J. M., and Iber, F. L.: Pulmonary function studies before and after jejunoileal bypass surgery. *Digest Dis, 21:*553, 1976.
32. Bray, G. A., Barry, R. E., Benfield, J. R., Castelnuovo-Tedesco, P., and Rodin, J.: Intestinal bypass surgery for obesity decreases food intake and taste preferences. *Am J Clin Nutr, 29:*779, 1976.
33. Mason, E. E.: Jejunoileal bypass. *Am J Clin Nutr, 29:*938, 1976.
34. Hermreck, A. S., Jewell, W. R., and Hardin, C. A.: Gastric bypass for morbid obesity: results and complications. *Surgery, 80:*498, 1976.
35. Stunkard, A. J.: Environment and obesity: recent advances in our understanding of regulation of food intake in man. *Fed Proc, 27:*1367, 1968.
36. Garrow, J. S.: Diet and obesity. *Proc R Soc Med, 66:*642, 1973.
37. Kempner, W., Newborg, B. C., Peschel, H. L., and Skyler, J. S.: Treatment of massive obesity with rice/reduction diet program. An analysis of 106 patients with at least a 45-kg. weight loss. *Arch Intern Med, 135:*1575, 1975.
38. Paulsen, B. K., Lutz, R. N., McReynolds, W. T., and Kohrs, M. B.: Behavior therapy for weight control: long-term results of two programs with nutritionists as therapists. *Am J Clin Nutr, 29:*880, 1976.
39. Mok, M. S., Parker, L. N., Voina, S., and Bray, G. A.: Treatment of obesity by acupuncture. *Am J Clin Nutr, 29:*832, 1976.
40. Stein, M. R., Julis, R. E., Peck, C. C., Hinshaw, W., Sawicki, J. E., and Deller, J. J., Jr.: Ineffectiveness of human chorionic gonadotropin in weight reduction: a double-blind study. *Am J Clin Nutr, 29:*940, 1976.
41. Garrow, J. S.: *Energy Balance and Obesity in Man.* Amsterdam, North Holland Publishing Co., 1974.
42. Miller, D. S., and Mumford, P.: Gluttony, 1. An experimental study of overeating low- or high-protein diets. *Am J Clin Nutr, 20:*1212, 1967.
43. Miller, D. S., Mumford, P., and Stock, M. J.: Gluttony, 2. Thermogenesis in overeating man. *Am J Clin Nutr, 20:*1223, 1967.
44. Felsher, B. F.: Effect of changes in dietary components on the serum bilerubin in Gilbert's syndrome. *Am J Clin Nutr, 29:*705, 1976.

PROTEIN

ALTHOUGH PROTEIN IS often referred to only as a substance responsible for the body's structure, its other roles in the human economy are both diverse and important. For one thing, all enzymes are proteins, and no biochemical functions are conceivable without them. Life as we know it depends on enzymes. However, even in severe protein deficiency, intracellular enzyme function is maintained despite large losses of protein. This is true because a decrease in intracellular enzyme activity does not become physiologically significant until the diminution amounts to 90 percent or more. Some, but not all, hormones are protein or constituents of proteins. The exceptions are the steroidal hormones—the sex and adrenocortical hormones. Parathormone, insulin, glucagon, the gastrins, angiotensin, certain newly recognized, smooth-muscle-regulating hormones, secretin, etc. are all peptides. The pituitary trophic hormones and the hypothalamic releasing factors are all peptides also. Unlike the enzymes, relatively small changes in hormone activity may cause symptoms. Some of the most rapidly acting hormones are derivatives of tyrosine (thyroxine, catecholamines) or tryptophan (serotonin, melatonin). Polymers of catecholamines and of dihydroxyphenylalamine (dopa) are precursors of melanin, not only in the skin, but in the brain, heart, and liver. It is evident that to consider proteins as mere structural elements is grossly misleading. Nevertheless, except for the decrease in some pituitary hormones in starvation, protein depletion in degrees encountered in our country reveals itself in adults only by emaciation and by edema due to hypoalbuminemia. In growing children and in pregnant women, protein depletion can have much more serious manifestations. Of course, the growth requirements of children and adolescents divert an increased percent of the dietary protein to building up tissues and their supply of enzymes.

Protein has, in addition, an important role in intermediary

16

metabolism. It serves as a source of carbohydrate to provide energy for intracellular processes. After amino acids are de-aminated, the residue (about 58% of the total weight) is meta-bolized as carbohydrate. Since the body's glycogen stores are not large, they are rapidly exhausted when carbohydrate is needed, and under these circumstances body proteins contribute to the carbohydrate pool through the process of gluconeogenesis.

Much money and effort have been expended in studies of protein nutrition designed to define necessary and optimal intakes both in an absolute sense and also in relation to total caloric intake.[1-5] This literature has been reviewed by Garza et al.[5] It appears that nitrogen requirements are increased at low levels of calorie intake.[5] The methods used to study nitrogen balance in man are notable for their possibilities of error in calcula-tion and interpretation. For one thing, using the twenty-four-hour urine creatinine output as a stable indicator of the adequacy of urine collections in balance studies is not valid.[6] The ambiguities are such as to lead some authors[7] to conclude that egg protein is not an efficient source of nitrogen. Actually, egg protein, like all other good-quality proteins, is less well utilized at requirement levels than at deficiency levels. Some proteins show even greater differences in this regard. The relation between energy intake and protein intake cannot be dismissed. One method currently used to determine protein requirements is to give the subjects a protein-free diet and study their nitrogen output in urine and stool (called "obligatory nitrogen losses"). This method seems to show that this loss in relation to body weight is independent of age.[8] However, there are large interindividual variations as calculated by this as well as other methods.[4, 8] This markedly difficult, obscure, and complicated field may yet become clarified through the meticulous studies of the Massachusetts Institute of Technology group[2, 8] and others, but that day is not yet in sight, and at the moment precise recommendations cannot be made.*

---

* These matters are beyond the interest of most clinicians, but those who want to know about them should read Garza, C., Scrimshaw, N. S., and Young, V. R.: Human protein requirements: a long-term metabolic nitrogen study in young men to evaluate the 1976 FAO/WHO safe level of protein intake. *J Nutr,* *107*:335, 1977. The data of this elegant study throw doubt on the validity of the conclusions of the FAO/WHO study. Moreover, the findings show discrepancies

There are data that suggest that protein intakes of 0.4 grams per kilogram of body weight per day are adequate. Thus, a healthy man weighing 70 kilograms would be in balance with an intake of 25 to 28 grams of protein per day—that is, with a calorie intake of around 100 to 115 per day from protein. Some recent current calculations show that theoretically it is enough to obtain 3 or 4 percent of calories from high quality protein, or 4 to 6 percent if the protein taken is not completely utilizable. This is consistent with the aforementioned intake of 25 to 28 grams of protein per day by a 70 kilogram man. However, the actual data from all over the world[4] show that the intake of calories from protein is usually 12 to 14 percent of the total, only rarely falling to 10 percent or lower. In Alaska it is 29 percent. It is clear that all over the world, except in famine areas, the populations take more protein than experts say is necessary. The theory is clearly wrong. The eating of protein has changed in the last fifty years. In many populations breads or other wheat products were a chief source of protein. The development of resistant strains of wheat was accompanied by a decrease of 50 percent of its protein content. Hence, the current large intake of protein is associated with an increase in the percentage of protein calories derived from animal protein— meat, fowl, fish, eggs, milk, cheese.

The reported figures for the average daily intake of meat in this country are difficult to interpret since, until recently, the reports were based solely on the total carcass weight of the slaughtered animals. About 50 percent of a steer and 43 percent of a hog are not used for human food. Moreover, the meat served as food contains bone and gristle that are not eaten and fat that is not eaten or is drained away in cooking. It appears that the average American eats less than 3 ounces a day of lean meat, fowl, or fish. This seems low when compared to the FDA recommendation of two or more feedings weighing 4 to 6 ounces of these proteins.

---

when nitrogen losses are calculated by three different methods, probably because the losses of nitrogen through the skin are three times as large as those assumed in earlier calculations.

Meticulous studies of this sort will, we hope, eventually remove the unrecognized ambiguities that underlie some current official recommendations.

The utilization of the nitrogen in the protein depends on at least three dietary factors. One is the total intake of protein in food. Persons who have a relatively low protein intake utilize their protein more efficiently than those with a high intake.[1, 3] Aside from the fact that this increased metabolic efficiency is manifested at the amino acid level, little is known about the phenomenon. Urea may be reabsorbed from the bladder, and we know from studies in uremia that urea can enter the metabolic pool. In addition, another phenomenon affects the utilization of ingested protein, the so-called "protein-sparing" effect of food eaten with the protein. Available data indicate that in normal persons carbohydrate does this better than fat, but the mechanism is unknown. Still another factor is the quality of the protein itself. Proteins vary in their ability to be utilized to carry out the functions that proteins have in the body. Some proteins are incomplete, i.e. lacking essential amino acids. The essential amino acids were recognized through studies in animals made several decades ago. Comparisons of intakes of intact proteins with the effects of their corresponding amino acids are difficult.[9, 10] Studies in man are difficult to carry out, and the data at hand are fragmentary.[11] However important these data are and will prove to be, they are as yet not able to serve as a directing force in human nutrition. For the most part the incomplete proteins are vegetable, a notable example being soy protein. Gelatin is an incomplete animal protein. A varied diet will provide all the essential amino acids.

Is there any harm associated with the worldwide supranormal intakes of protein? Evidently not. For one thing, the recommended requirement is for "almost all normal people"—whatever that means. Is a healthy person under some small and transient stress to be considered unhealthy? I think not. Yet it is a fact that stresses, either physical or mental, can cause large losses of nitrogen from the body. Scrimshaw[12] has summarized the older literature. Blackburn et al.[13] have added more recent references as well as new data. The nitrogen loss of stress is probably owing to gluconeogenesis instituted by adrenal corticoids. It is a complicated phenomenon, in which plasma and muscle amino acids are diverted to the liver, the urine loss of amino acids diminishing.[14] The loss of body protein that occurs in stress may have deleterious consequences, notably poor wound healing and, if long continued, loss of protein from the matrix of bone. Blackburn et al.[13] insist that part of the trouble is an excessive production of insulin brought out by the administration of dextrose in water, the insulin preventing utilization of body fat stores. Giving an amino acid mixture intravenously was reported to have remedied the situation. This view seemingly receives support from the observation that giving glucose alone does not suppress gluconeogenesis from amino acids in sepsis.[15] More recent studies confirm that glucose alone does not prevent protein loss in the postoperative period.[16] However, the mechanism is not that presented by Blackburn et al.;[13] the state of the lipid metabolism has little to do with the matter, and treating the protein loss of stress can be accomplished only by giving protein plus, of course, adequate calories. During severe febrile illnesses there are complicated changes in amino acid metabolism that have stimulated much theoretical discussion.[17, 18]

A question that arises frequently concerns the amount of protein that athletes need to attain maximal fitness. There is no definite answer, but 100 grams per day seems to be adequate despite large losses in sweating.[19] There is no reason to believe that activity changes the protein requirements significantly.

How is the physician to judge the adequacy of protein intake? Serum albumin measurements are of little value except in severe depletion. Attempts have been made to use examination of scalp hairs to detect protein malnutrition.[20] The validity and clinical usefulness of this approach remain to be established.

One usually ignored phenomenon that is associated with hypoalbuminemia in sick persons is the altered clearance of some medications owing to inadequate protein binding.[21]

Another question that must be faced is whether the intake of protein in amounts higher than officially recommended, especially animal protein, is harmful to man. At the moment a few authorities, using data from population studies, have begun to claim that eating meat causes colonic cancer. Aside from the impossibility of proving any etiology by any such studies, there are certain observations that cast doubt on the concept. These are the facts that there is no excess of colonic cancer in Alaskans, who eat considerably more meat than the rest of Americans, and colon cancer is less common in Mormons than in other Americans despite a higher intake of meat by the Mormons.[22]

RECOMMENDATIONS

In normal persons an intake of 70 to 100 grams of protein per day seems reasonable. The protein intake in patients under stress should be at least 125 grams per day. Those who show poor wound healing (including bedsores) as a result of protracted stress should receive as much as tolerable, using concentrated oral protein supplements. I have used as much as 200 grams per day. Of course, patients with renal or liver insufficiency cannot tolerate high intakes of protein.

REFERENCES

1. Waterlow, J. C.: Observations on the mechanism of adaptation to low protein intakes. *Lancet*, 2:1091, 1968.
2. Steffee, W. P., Goldsmith, R. S., Pencharz, P. B., Scrimshaw, N. S., and Young, V. R.: Dietary protein intake and dynamic aspects of whole body nitrogen metabolism in adult humans. *Metabolism*, 25:281, 1976.
3. Nicol, B. M. and Phillips, P. G.: Endogenous excretion and utilization of dietary protein. *Br J Nutr*, 35:181, 1976.
4. Beaton, G. H. and Swiss, L. D.: Evaluation of the nutritional quality of food supplies: prediction of "desirable" or "safe" protein: calorie ratios. *Am J Clin Nutr*, 27:485, 1974.
5. Garza, C., Scrimshaw, N. S., and Young, V. R.: Human protein requirements: the effect of variations in energy intake within the maintenance range. *Am J Clin Nutr*, 29:280, 1976.
6. Greenblatt, D. J., Ransel, B. J., Harmatz, J. S., Smith, T. W., Duhme, D. W., and Koch-Weser, J.: Variability of 24-hour creatinine excretion by normal subjects. *J Clin Pharmacol*, 16:321, 1976.
7. Calloway, D. H. and Margen, S.: Variations in endogenous nitrogen excretion and dietary nitrogen utilization as determinants of human protein requirement. *J Nutr*, 101:205, 1971.
8. Scrimshaw, N. S., Perera, W. D. A., and Young, V. R.: Protein requirements of man: obligatory urinary and fecal nitrogen losses in women. *J Nutr*, 106:665, 1976.
9. Clark, H. E., Moon, W-H., Bailey, L. B., and Panemangelore, M.: Nitrogen retention and plasma amino acids of adults who consumed

isonitrogenous diets containing rice and milk or wheat versus their constituent animo acids. *Am J Clin Nutr,* 29:1343, 1976.

10. Bailey, L. B. and Clark, H. E.: Plasma amino acids and nitrogen retention of human subjects who consumed isonitrogenous diets containing rice and wheat or their constituent amino acids with and without additional lysine. *Am J Clin Nutr,* 29:1353, 1976.

11. Swendseid, M. E. and Koppler, J. E.: Nitrogen balance, plasma amino acid levels and amino acid requirements. *Trans NY Acad Sci,* 25:471, 1973.

12. Scrimshaw, N. S.: Nutrition and Stress. In G. E. W. Wolstenholme (Ed.): *Diet and Bodily Constitution.* Boston, Little Brown and Co., 1964.

13. Blackburn, G. L., Flatt, J. P., Clowes, C. H. A., O'Donnell, T. F., and Hensle, T. E.: Protein sparing therapy during periods of starvation with sepsis or trauma. *Ann Surg,* 177:588, 1973.

14. Wannemacher, R. W., Dinterman, R. E., Pekarek, R. S., Bartelloni, P. J., and Beisel, W. R.: Urinary amino acid excretion during experimentally induced sandfly fever in man. *Am J Clin Nutr,* 28:110, 1975.

15. Long, C. L., Kinney, J. M., and Guger, J. W.: Nonsuppressability of gluconeogenesis by glucose in septic patients. *Metabolism,* 25:190, 1976.

16. Greenberg, G. R., Marlis, E. B., Anderson, G. H., Langer, B., Spence, W., Tover, E. B., and Jeejeebhoy, K. N.: Protein-sparing therapy in postoperative patients. Effects of added hypocaloric glucose or lipid. *N Engl J Med,* 294:1411, 1976.

17. O'Donnell, T. F., Jr., Clowes, G. H. A., Jr., Blackburn, G. L., Ryan, N. T., Benotti, P. N., and Miller, J. D. B.: Proteolysis associated with a deficit of peripheral energy fuel substrates in septic man. *Surgery* 80:192, 1976.

18. Wannemacher, R. W., Klainer, A. S., Dinterman, R. E., and Beisel, W. R.: The significance of an increased serum phenylalanine-tyrosine ratio during infection. *Am J Clin Nutr,* 29:997, 1976.

19. Consalazio, C. F., Johnson, H. L., Nelson, R. A., Dramise, J. G., and Shala, J. H.: Protein metabolism during intensive physical training in the young adult. *Am J Clin Nutr,* 28:29, 1975.

20. Jordan, V. E.: Protein status of the elderly as measured by dietary intake, hair tissue, and serum albumin. *Am J Clin Nutr,* 29:522, 1976.

21. Thiessen, J. J., Sellers, E. M., Denbeigh, P., and Dolman, L.: Plasma protein binding of diazepam and tolbutamide in chronic alcoholics. *J Clin Pharmacol,* 16:345, 1976.

22. Lyon, J. L., Klauber, M. R., Gardner, J. W., and Smart, C. R.: Cancer incidence in Mormons and non-Mormons in Utah, 1966-1970. *N Engl J Med,* 294:129, 1976.

CARBOHYDRATES

ALTHOUGH MOST LAYMEN and some others are accustomed to consider all dietary carbohydrates as essentially similar, there are important metabolic differences between the various categories. The only consistent similarity they share is their calorie value, slightly over 4 per gram.

The carbohydrates in food consist mainly of the complex polysaccharides, starch and glycogen, and the disaccharides, sucrose and lactose. Carbohydrates in food yield about 50 percent of the calories ingested by man. However, it must be remembered that, in addition, 58 percent of the ingested protein is, after digestion and deamination, metabolized like carbohydrate. It is evident, therefore, that carbohydrate is the main source of energy in man. There are other small saccharides in legumes that may be eaten in large amounts, but they cannot be digested or absorbed. They may, however, be acted upon by intestinal bacteria, with the production of large amounts of gas.

The two complex polysaccharides in our food, starch and cellulose, are similar in one respect but markedly different in another. Starch, whatever its source, is a polymer made up of glucose elements. An analogous structure is found in cellulose, but the linkages are enough different to make cellulose indigestible. When starch is ingested, the action of duodenal amylopectin breaks it down into the disaccharide, maltose, plus the trisaccharide, maltobiose, plus the pectins which are polymers of five to a dozen glucose entities. The intestinal epithelium contains enzymes—the oligosaccharidases—that split all these compounds to glucose. Thus sucrose-isomaltase splits sucrose to glucose and fructose, and dextrin to glucose; and alpha-glucosidase splits maltose and maltobiose to glucose. Lactase splits lactose to glucose and galactose.

Since glucose is the sole end product of starch digestion and is also released in the digestion of sucrose and lactose, glucose comprises about 80 percent of the carbohydrate absorbed from the intestine. The monosaccharides are too large to be absorbed by diffusion, and the intestine contains transport mechanisms for this purpose.

In a variety of malabsorption syndromes, the intestinal lining may be so changed as to be unable either to make the oligosaccharidases or to maintain the transport mechanisms. Accordingly, the well-known symptoms develop. The same is true in cases of congenital enzyme deficiencies, e.g. lactase deficiency. The undigested and unabsorbed small saccharides act osmotically, drawing fluid into the lumen and initiating cramps, noisy guts, and diarrhea. Bacteria may attack the unabsorbed sugars, producing gas and the consequent bloating and flatulence. These disorders do not lie within the province of this work.

The main role of sugars in the economy of the body is to provide energy. One sugar, lactose, has additional functions. Its role in enhancing calcium absorption is well known, although not understood. Lactose is also believed to enhance protein absorption, but this has not been demonstrated in man. One of the two constituents of lactose is galactose. This sugar is a constituent of brain lipids but apparently the brain synthesizes it and the diet is not its source.

Arrangements for storing unused carbohydrate as such are notably inadequate. Some glucose is repolymerized to glycogen in the liver, but the amount is not large, and it is easily exhausted when intake falls. There is also an accumulation of glycogen in red muscle, but this is for the use of muscles and is broken down to pyruvate (and lactate) during exertion. The unused excess is carried to the liver to become hepatic glycogen. Since glucose, when taken in excess, cannot be stored as carbohydrate, and certainly not as protein, it is stored as fat. The formation of lipid from sugar can, of course, occur in the liver, but its occurrence in adipose tissue is perhaps more interesting. Here the rate of transformation of glucose to lipid varies as the size of the fat cell.[1] Since in obesity the fat cells are increased, not in number but in size, it is apparent that obesity owing to increased carbohydrate intake is self-perpetuating and perhaps self-accelerating. The decreased utilization of calories for heat production in obesity has been noted (page 6).

The regulation of blood sugar level and the relation of hunger to it is too complicated and too incompletely known to define at present. Insulin is, of course, essential for the utilization of glucose, although its mechanism of action is not totally understood. Some authors[2] favor the idea that glucagon is a factor that participates in the regulation of blood glucose level by opposing the action of insulin. However, others oppose this view.[3, 4] Certainly infusing glucagon into an arm artery has no effect on the metabolism of the muscle or fat tissue in the arm[5] and, hence, does not seem to play any role in cellular carbohydrate metabolism. Whatever the deficiencies in our appreciation of the details of glucose metabolism, physicians must still deal with clinical problems that seem to be associated with it.

One condition that should be appreciated is so-called "starvation diabetes."[6, 7] Patients starved completely or given a very low carbohydrate diet develop a diabetic type of glucose tolerance curve. This is not due to depressed utilization of glucose by peripheral tissues.[7] The insulin rise on feeding glucose after starvation is slow and prolonged, resembling that seen in diabetes mellitus.[6, 7] The blood free fatty acid, acetoacetate, and beta-hydroxybutyrate levels rise in starvation and fall when glucose is given. The serum lactate level also falls after glucose.[7] However, the diabetic type of glucose tolerance curve need not occur in all persons on a low carbohydrate intake if they are healthy and if the diet is not too high in fat.[8] (Protein was given to make up for the calories of the excluded carbohydrates.) In starvation, the serum glucagon level rises markedly, although it falls somewhat after a time. Actually, the mechanism of "starvation diabetes" is not known, for although the glucagon output rises, this is not now believed to cause a diabetic glucose tolerance curve.

When persons with true reactive hypoglycemia are given a low carbohydrate diet, their glucose tolerance deteriorates to a degree much worse than occurs in normal persons.[8] Giving persons with this type of hypoglycemia a high protein diet aborts the reactive hypoglycemia, although the glucose tolerance is not as good as before the protein is given.[8]*

---

* For a scholarly biochemical discussion of hypoglycemia the reader is referred to Permutt, M. A.: Postprandial hypoglycemia. *Diabetes*, 25:720, 1976.

One syndrome that is commonly called hypoglycemia is actually not hypoglycemia. An error is often owing to poorly performed glucose tolerance tests. In some cases, due to the patient's apprehension, the initial level is falsely high. As the patient relaxes during the hours that the test occupies, the basal level falls so that when the test ends, a blood concentration of glucose is reached that is 20 or 30 milligrams percent below the erroneous "control" level. A diagnosis of "hypoglycemia" then seems established. To carry out the test correctly, the patient should be given a very high carbohydrate intake for three days. On the day of the test, the patient must rest in bed for half an hour before the first blood specimen is taken. To be perfectly certain of having a valid reading, a second fasting specimen may be taken fifteen or twenty minutes after the first. When carried out carefully, the test usually reveals a normal glucose tolerance curve in such patients. The laboratory error, nevertheless, does not explain their symptoms: they do have weaknesses, etc. a few hours after eating a carbohydrate meal. In some of the cases studied this is owing to a block in the utilization of pyruvate, a breakdown product of glucose. Only 20 percent of the energy derived from glucose is released when glucose becomes pyruvate. The other 80 percent develops when the pyruvate is metabolized in the Krebs cycle, ultimately to carbon dioxide and water. When a block in pyruvate utilization occurs, much of the energy is lost or, if delivered, becomes available so slowly as to be unnoticed. Hence, symptoms suggestive of hypoglycemia in some patients may be present without an abnormal blood glucose curve. It should be noted that alcohol, or rather its primary metabolite, acetaldehyde, circumvents this block and will relieve the symptoms, as some patients learn to their ultimate detriment. Actually, patients with this pseudohypoglycemic syndrome feel better if most of their dietary sugar is replaced with protein. Although this enters the metabolic pool slowly, it does so for a much longer period than does sugar and, hence, is likely to sustain them better. It is probable that patients of the sort just described are laboring under some form of stress. Their abnormally slow utilization of pyruvate can be reproduced in normal people by giving them epinephrine in amounts too small to affect the pulse and blood pressure. Adrenocorticotropic hormone (ACTH) or adrenal corticoids will also reproduce the abnormality in normal persons.[9]

The disturbed carbohydrate metabolism associated with a variety of stresses has been known for many decades. Dozens of papers have recorded stress hyperglycemia and glycosuria. Clinicians have long been aware that fevers, trauma, or vascular accidents aggravate diabetes or make it overt when it is latent. Small children may develop phenomenally high blood sugar levels with fevers and yet afterwards show no sign of disturbed sugar metabolism. Almost all the published reports refer simply to blood glucose levels, but some mention also intermediary metabolites. (All these data have been collected, with much added material, in a paper that has the somewhat misleading title *Carbohydrate Metabolism in Mental Disease.*[9]) The disorder of intermediary metabolism, recognized by sluggishness in the utilization of pyruvic and other keto acids, occurs in many different kinds of stress states, for the body does not distinguish the quality of stress, only the intensity. The biochemical pattern also has been found in metabolic disorders such as thiamine deficiency, hyperthyroidism, and hepatic failure, and in some women who take oral contraceptives. The mechanism is not known, although some authorities believe that the disorder resides in the malate enzyme of the Krebs cycle.

Additional studies have been made in recent years, and they point to gluconeogenesis as an important part of the process. Studies in subhuman primates[10, 11] have shown that myocardial infarctions, sepsis, and trauma cause an outpouring of glucagon. Serum growth hormone and insulin levels remain normal, but there is an excessive rise in serum insulin after glucose is given. In man a similar increase in gluconeogenesis has been found after myocardial infarctions[12] and infection[13, 14] and trauma.[14] Here too the glucagon output has been found increased, whereas serum growth hormone and insulin levels remain unchanged.[12] Giving glucose does not suppress the increased gluconeogenesis from alamine[13] and from fat.[14] It is important to remember that the best treatment for the metabolic disorder of stress is not the sweet drinks we have been accustomed to recommend but, instead, easily digested protein, such as, perhaps, chicken soup.

The effect of different carbohydrates on blood sugar and serum insulin has been studied. Giving sugar in a meal causes a much lower rise than when given in a drink.[15] Rice causes much lower rises than potato.[15] Giving fiber with the carbohydrate, i.e. guar or pectin, lowers the blood levels markedly.[16] The effects seem to be related to the speeds of digestion and absorption.

Several additional topics relating to carbohydrate metabolism remain to be covered. One is the matter of endurance. This problem is largely one of carbohydrate metabolism in periods of short but extreme effort, as recent discussions have emphasized.[17] However, the storage of carbohydrate in muscles is not easily manipulated.

Another topic much in the public eye, if not mind, is the possible role of diet in atherosclerosis. One hypothesis, neither more nor less valid than any of the others, holds that the cause is sucrose. Ahrens recently reviewed the large but unconvincing literature on this subject[18] and raised questions about the purported relation of sucrose ingestion to atherosclerosis.

Unfortunately, carbohydrate as made available for ingestion in this country has been largely depleted of vitamins, minerals, and fiber. These should be taken in adequate amounts as discussed elsewhere in this book (See pages 77, 96, and 167). In our culture the easy availability of carbohydrate foods may lead to their intake in excessive amounts. This may lead to obesity with its complications and to deficiencies of certain vitamins and minerals. This is especially likely to occur if the foods are highly processed. An extreme example is offered by the sugar used as a food sweetener. It is a chemical triumph but a nutritional hazard.

RECOMMENDATIONS

The normal intake of carbohydrate amounts to about 50 percent of the total calories. There is no evidence that a lower carbohydrate intake is harmful.

Choose carbohydrate food sold in boxes carefully. Those that have been stripped of their naturally occurring vitamins and minerals should be avoided.

REFERENCES

1. Harrison, F. C. and King-Roach, A. D.: Cell size and glucose oxidation rate in adipose tissue from non-diabetic and diabetic obese human subjects. *Clin Sci Mol Med, 50*:171, 1976.
2. Gerich, J. E., Lorenzi, M., Hane, S., Gustafson, G., Guillemin, R., and Forsham, P. N.: Evidence for a physiologic role of pancreatic glucagon in human glucose hemeostasis: studies with somatostatin. *Metabolism, 24*:175, 1975.
3. Sherwin, R. S., Fisher, M., Hendler, R., and Felig, P.: Hyperglucagonemia and blood glucose regulation in normal, obese, and diabetic subjects. *N Engl J Med, 294*:455, 1976.
4. Levine, R.: Glucagon and the regulation of blood sugar. *N Engl J Med, 294*:495, 1976.
5. Pozefsky, T., Tancredi, R. G., Moxley, R. T., Dupre, J., and Tobian, J. D.: Metabolism of forearm tissues in man. Studies with glucagon. *Diabetes, 25*:128, 1976.
6. Unger, R. H., Eisentrant, A. M., and Madison, L. L.: The effects of total starvation upon the levels of circulating glucagon and insulin in man. *J Clin Invest, 42*:1051, 1963.
7. Jackson, R. A., Advani, U., Perry, G., Rogers, J., Peters, N., Day, S., and Pilkington, T. R. E.: Dietary diabetes. The influence of a low carbohydrate diet on forearm metabolism in man. *Diabetes, 22*:145, 1973.
8. Anderson, J. W. and Herman, R. N.: Effects of carbohydrate restriction on glucose tolerance of normal men and reactive hypoglycemic patients. *Am J Clin Nutr, 28*:748, 1975, with addendum on p. 1339.
9. Altschule, M. D.: Carbohydrate metabolism in mental disease; associated changes in phosphate metabolism. In Himwich, H. E. (Ed.): *Biochemistry, Schizophrenia and the Affective Illnesses.* Baltimore, Williams and Wilkins Co., 1971, p. 333.
10. Bloom, S. R., Daniel, P. M., Johnston, D. I., Ogawa, O., and Pratt, O. E.: Release of glucagon induced by stress. *Q J Exp Physiol, 58*:99, 1973.
11. Geogre, D. T., Rayfield, E. J., and Wannemacher, R. W.: Altered glucoregulatory hormones during acute pneumococcal sepsis in the Rhesus monkey. *Diabetes, 25*:544, 1974.
12. Laniado, S., Segal, P., and Eshig, B.: The role of glucagon hypersecretion in the pathogenesis of hyperglycemia following myocardial infarction. *Circulation, 48*:797, 1973.
13. Long, C. L., Kinney, J. M., and Geiger, J. W.: Nonsuppressability of gluconeogenesis by glucose in septic patients. *Metabolism, 25*:193, 1976.
14. Blackburn, G. L., Flatt, J. P., Clowes, G. H. A., Jr., O'Donnell, T. F.,

and Hensle, T. E.: Protein sparing therapy during periods of starvation with sepsis or trauma. *Ann Surg, 177*:588, 1973.

15. Crapo, P. A., Reaven, G., and Olefsky, J.: Plasma glucose and insulin responses to orally administered simple and complex carbohydrates. *Diabetes, 25*:741, 1976.

16. Jenkins, D. J. A., Goff, D. V., Leeds, A. R., Alberti, K. G. M. M., Woleven, T. M. S., Gassull, M. A., and Hochaday, T. D. R.: Unabsorbable carbohydrates and diabetes: decreased postprandial hyperglycemia. *Lancet, 2*:172, 1976.

17. Lewis, S. and Gutin, B.: Nutrition and endurance. *Am J Clin Nutr, 26*:1011, 1973.

18. Ahrens, R. A.: Sucrose, hypertension, and heart disease: an historical perspective. *Am J Clin Nutr, 27*:403, 1974.

FAT

Fᴀᴛ ɪꜱ ᴀ ᴍᴏꜱᴛ important part of the diet. Not only does the fat in meat and fish constitute a necessary source of flavor, but butterfat, either as such or as cream, is commonly added to grains and other vegetables to add flavor. Dietary fat also has essential physiologic roles. It delays emptying of the stomach, thereby delaying the onset of hunger, and stimulates the emptying of the gallbladder, providing essential materials for the absorption of fat-soluble vitamins and other dietary elements.

The various body lipids participate in functions and processes much more diverse and complicated than do protein and carbohydrates. They provide gross structural elements of nervous tissues, and, at the other end of the scale, they are part of every cell membrane and subcellular membrane. In the form of adipose tissue, they store energy as glycerol—or cholesterol-esters for years or, again, provide free fatty acids for quick use in energy-demanding functions. When glucose utilization is impaired, as in starvation, very high fat intake, or diabetes, this energy-providing role is enhanced. Catecholamines cause the release of free fatty acids from adipose tissue, as do a variety of stresses.

Fats are ingested as such, or made in the body from carbohydrate or from portions of amino acids. When cells are injured in some ways they are likely to cut down their synthesis of protein and manufacture instead large amounts of lipids. The utility of this last process is not evident. Indeed there is reason to believe that it may be harmful, a reality that must be taken into account in studying disease processes but which regrettably usually is not.

A vast amount of literature on the metabolism of fat has accumulated in the past few years. It is not enough, for there are many gaps in our knowledge. One can say not only that fat metabolism is not well understood, but that in some ways it is misunderstood.

The clinical significance of the blood triglyceride concentrations in disease is not clear. These substances increase in the blood in obesity due to overeating, but in this circumstance their concentration may be lowered by exercise (see pages 5-12). On the other hand, they rise when renal insufficiency produces retention of nitrogenous products, and they rise even more with dialysis, but this seems not to be related to the diet.[1] There seems to be a deficiency of lipolytic enzyme activity in uremia.

There has been a major controversy about the relation of specific carbohydrates to hypertriglyceridemia. In one study, eating of up to 300 grams of sucrose a day did raise the blood triglyceride levels, whereas eating this much starch food did not.[2] This sucrose intake is so far outside the range of normal experience as to make the validity of the data seem dubious. With more reasonable amounts of any type of carbohydrate—sucrose, starch, fruit, legume, or vegetable—no change in serum triglyceride level occurs.[3] (Nevertheless there are diseases of triglyceride metabolism, which are not considered here, in which carbohydrate in moderate amounts does cause worsening.)

Estrogen raises the plasma triglyceride level, and this change is enhanced by progestins.[4] Although the increases may be cyclic, a considerable number of women, those who take oral contraceptives and those who take estrogen after menopause, must have persistently high triglyceride levels in the blood.

Some authors, a minority, have published statistics that seem to show a correlation between the occurrence of coronary atherosclerosis and serum triglyceride levels. Other authors find no such relation. The conclusion that elevation of serum triglyceride level will cause atherosclerosis has little to support it. This applies to familial hypertriglyceridemia as well as other types.[5] However, patients with familial combined hyperlipidemia, which is accompanied by hypertriglyceridemia alone or combined with hypercholesterolemia, or by neither of these changes, may have more coronary atherosclerosis than the normal population for reasons not at all evident.[5]

The matter of essential fatty acids should be mentioned. Strictly speaking there is only one, arachidonic acid, but it is made so easily in the body from linoleic acid that the two together bear the designation. Linoleic acid is so widespread

in nature that a deficiency of essential fatty acids, well known
in experimental animals, is rare in man. Since the deficiency will
not occur if these fatty acids make up 1 percent of the calories
taken, it is difficult to produce it. It occurs in sick infants given
fat-free intravenous feedings for even short periods[6] and may be
so induced in adult man also.[7] It is hardly likely that most
practitioners will ever encounter an instance of it, but they
should be aware of it.

Another blood constituent, the phospholipids, has been studied
in relation to diet, but the data obtained do not help us in our
understanding of the general nutritional problems under discussion in this work.

To some extent the same can be said about cholesterol. The
volume of writings about cholesterol is very great, but the
usable information about this substance is small.

Cholesterol is ubiquitous in animal cells. Animal life without
cholesterol is unimaginable. However, its role in bodily function
has never been understood, and today biochemists refer to
cholesterol as a most mysterious substance. Some of its functions
are known: it is a precursor substance needed for the manufacture of the sex hormones and of the adrenal cortex hormones
that regulate many phases of salt, sugar, protein, and fat metabolism in the animal body. During exercise, cholesterol can serve
as a source of energy and is oxidized to carbon dioxide and
water just as any other source of energy, such as sugar and fat,
is oxidized. However, in the main its functions have not been
elucidated. The prevailing belief is that within each body cell
cholesterol is present as part of the cell membranes and intracellular membranes that determine the transport into, in, and
out of the cells of all the nutrients and all the waste products.
The very origin of the cells' cholesterol is mysterious. Part of
the cholesterol in the body comes from the food taken in, but
more of it is manufactured in the body. This, too, is mysterious,
because cholesterol is a large and complicated molecule, and
animal cells cannot manufacture such molecules—except for
cholesterol. (Plants can manufacture molecules of extraordinary
complexity and, hence, in this respect at least, might be considered
biologically superior to animals.) Cholesterol rarely, if ever,
exists in a free state in normal animal cells or in the tissue fluids

or the blood plasma. It is combined with various proteins and a number of other substances to form the lipoproteins. Cholesterol (in combined forms) is a significant nutrient constituent of many foods, such as eggs, milk products, and meats.

When body cells are subjected to adverse conditions or to disease processes, they seem to prepare themselves for bad times by changing the chemical state of their contents and by storing up substances that might be needed. These include various carbohydrates and fatty substances. Thus, when a body cell is forced to live in an unhealthy or otherwise abnormal environment, it responds by changing the chemical state of its fat, so that it becomes visible, and then manufactures more fat—including cholesterol—to store against hard times.

The fact that cholesterol is a mysterious substance not only permits, but encourages, speculation concerning its effects and properties. This has led to an enormous proliferation of medical writings that express a variety of ideas concerning the subject. One of the ideas current in this country is that eating cholesterol (or other substances that are said to interact with cholesterol, such as saturated fats) causes the atherosclerosis responsible for heart attacks, strokes, and so forth. This notion has no substantial backing; that is, whatever data have been brought forward to support it are found, on examination, either not to support it or to contradict it. This is not the place to argue the etiology of atherosclerosis—it has been discussed in detail elsewhere.[8, 9, 10] Our only purpose here is to consider the available data bearing on the possible role of nutritional factors in causing it. This discussion will recognize that diet is important in the treatment of precursor conditions such as hypertension (low salt), diabetes (controlled sugar), and obesity (low calories), but these do not apply directly to the atherosclerosis itself.

There is no doubt that in many of the populations studied there is a parallel between serum cholesterol level and the likelihood of having a myocardial infarction above the age of thirty and more strikingly above the age of forty. There are, however, exceptions in which elevated serum cholesterol levels are not necessarily associated with coronary artery disease. The serum cholesterol level relative to that of others of similar age seems to be determined for each person by the early twenties.[12] It is interesting to note that in this study the average serum cholesterol level rose by over 31 percent in nineteen years, but the rank order of the individual subjects remained almost the same. (None developed evidence of coronary atherosclerosis.) This was a good study, as it allowed for the effects of apprehension and for seasonal variations. The latter may be large. Some surprising data have been published. The fact that about 35 percent of children in two European studies were found to have high serum cholesterol values[14] is inexplicable. Breast-fed children do have higher serum cholesterol levels than bottle-fed, but this difference disappears by the age of one year.[15]

What have elevated serum cholesterol levels to do with diet? Certainly the intake of saturated fat, including saturated fat of animal origin, does not cause it, to cite only some recent studies.[16-20] Nevertheless, the taking of a diet low in animal protein is widely recommended in this country as a sure preventive of heart attacks.

Since eating animal protein and saturated fat does not raise the serum cholesterol level or increase the incidence of coronary atherosclerosis,[8, 9, 10, 11, 17, 18] attention has turned in other directions, i.e. attempts to lower serum cholesterol levels by adding something to the diet. One is to add nicotinic acid in large amounts, but this has not been popular. Another is to add vegetable fiber; it has long been known that pectins in the diet lower serum cholesterol levels, but other vegetable fibers do not.[21] The introduction into the diet of large amounts of polyunsaturated fat is now strongly advocated and is supported by massive commercial advertising campaigns. Even nursing mothers have been told to take polyunsaturated fat in order to lower the serum cholesterol levels of their babies.[22] (As was pointed out previously, bottle-fed babies have low serum cholesterol levels.) There is no doubt that this diet will lower the serum cholesterol level by about 15 percent, but there is no evidence that it affects the incidence and severity of atherosclerosis, coronary or other. Some of the potential hazards of diets high in polyunsaturated acids were noted some time ago.[8] It causes the depletion of vitamin E stores as has again been emphasized.[23] In recent years an increased incidence of cancer in persons taking this diet has been noted.[24] This statistical finding might be considered merely one more of the wonderfully weird conclusions that statistical medicine seems to lead to if it were not for the fact that peroxidized polyunsaturated fatty acids do produce a carcinogen.[25]

The whole problem of serum cholesterol and atherosclerosis was put in a new light when a recent study, like a dozen others neglected during the last twenty-five years, showed that the amount of cholesterol carried in the blood attached to small proteins was *negatively* correlated with the incidence of atherosclerosis; that is, on a statistical basis, this cholesterol seemed to protect against atherosclerosis.[26] Of course it does not protect against atherosclerosis, but it should give food for thought to those who claim that cholesterol causes atherosclerosis.

What then is the relation of the common finding of a high serum cholesterol level and atherosclerosis? The answer seems to be that damaged arteries make cholesterol and pour it into the bloodstream.[27] High serum cholesterol levels are a symptom, not a cause, of atherosclerosis.

This discussion applies to native, i.e. unprocessed, cholesterol in foods. There is evidence that processed cholesterol, as in dried egg powder or dried whole milk powder, contains oxides of cholesterol that are demonstrably atherogenic.[9, 10] Since almost all commercially baked breads and cakes, as well as other commercially prepared foods, are made with these processed cholesterol-containing foods, the likelihood of atherosclerosis showing up as a disease of civilization, or at least industrialization, is very high.

Several other items must be considered. For example, some recent publications ascribe the occurrence of cancer of the colon to the production of carcinogens through the action of bacteria on fecal bile acids.[28, 29] The conclusion that colon cancer is caused by eating beef fat has been derived from these findings. It seems premature, for the statistics that purport to show a high incidence of colon cancer in meat eaters have not been validated (see page 20).

Another subject to be considered is what the consumption of processed vegetable fats might do. For one thing, those who use the so-called "nondairy" cream substitutes in order to avoid saturated fatty acids are in fact getting saturated fatty acids.[30]

The significance of this fact cannot be stated, since there is no substantial evidence that saturated fatty acids are harmful or that unsaturated fatty acids are beneficial. However, the metabolic fate of processed—usually hydrogenated—vegetable fats in the body is not completely known. In reported studies subjects who took hydrogenated vegetable fats ended with the same serum concentrations of cholesterol and triglycerides as those who took the unsaturated.[31] Nevertheless, the processed vegetable fats contain molecules whose shapes are so changed as to make it unlikely that they can be utilized normally to produce the energy we expect of fats. They do enter the various tissues that normally contain fatty acids, but their fate thereafter is not clear.[32] If not normally utilizable, to what extent do they accumulate? If accumulating, can they be used in times of need or will they merely occupy space? These questions will have to be answered.

The possibility that plant sterols may contribute to xanthomatosis, despite the fact that the fatty tumors consist mainly of cholesterol,[33] is an intriguing one.

RECOMMENDATIONS

There is no need to fear native fats. They should be eaten for energy and for appetite control. A current belief holds that an excess of fat, by causing ketosis, is harmful. Nevertheless, ketosis was regularly induced in the treatment of epilepsy some decades ago, with no evident harm. The intake of processed vegetable oils may distort metabolism, but this is not proved. Polyunsaturated fats cause vitamin E deficiency. It is possible that some of them are carcinogenic, but this is not established.

The only atherogenic fats known are certain cholesterol oxides created during the manufacture of dried egg and dried whole milk powders.

REFERENCES

1. McCosh, E. J., Solangi, K., Rivers, J. M., and Goodman, A.: Hypertriglyceridemia in patients with chronic renal insufficiency. *Am J Clin Nutr, 28*:1036, 1975.
2. Naismith, D. J., Strock, A. L., and Yudkin, J.: Effects of changes in the proportions of dietary carbohydrates and in energy intakes on the

plasma lipid concentrations in healthy young men. *Nutr Metab,* 16:296, 1974.

3. Grande, F., Anderson, J. T., and Keys, A.: Sucrose and various carbohydrate-containing foods and serum lipids in man. *Am J Clin Nutr,* 27:1043, 1974.

4. Young, D. L. and Chan, P. L.: Effects of a progestogen and a sequential type oral contraceptive on plasma vitamin A, vitamin E, cholesterol, and triglycerides. *Am J Clin Nutr,* 28:686, 1975.

5. Brunzell, J. D., Schrott, H. G., Motulsky, A. G., and Bierman, E. L.: Myocardial infarction in the familial forms of hypertriglyceridemia. *Metabolism,* 25:313, 1976.

6. Paulsrud, J. R., Pensler, L., Whitten, C. F., Stewart, S., and Holman, R. T.: Essential fatty acid deficiency in infants induced by fat-free intravenous feeding. *Am J Clin Nutr,* 25:897, 1972.

7. Fleming, C. R., Smith, L. M., and Hodges, R. E.: Essential fatty acid deficiency in adults receiving total parenteral nutrition. *Am J Clin Nutr,* 29:976, 1976.

8. Altschule, M. D.: The uselessness of diet in the treatment of atherosclerosis. In Ingelfinger, F. J., Relman, A. S., and Finland M. (Eds.): *Controversy in Internal Medicine.* Philadelphia, W. B. Saunders Co., 1966, p. 69.

9. Altschule, M. D.: The etiology of atherosclerosis. *Med Clin North Am,* 58:397, 1974.

10. Altschule, M. D.: Updating the cholesterol-atherosclerosis controversy. *Primary Care, 1*:253, 1974.

11. Oliver, M. F., Nimmi, I. A., Cooke, M., Carlson, L. A., and Olsson, A. G.: Ischaemic heart disease and associated risk factors in 40-year old men in Edinburgh and Stockholm. *Eur J Clin Lab Med, 5*:507, 1975.

12. Clark, D. A., Allen, M. F., and Wilson, F. H., Jr.: USAFAM cardiovascular disease followup study: comparisons of serum lipid and lipoprotein levels. *Aerosp Med, 45*:1167, 1974.

13. Werko, L.: Serum lipids in adult males. *Am J Clin Nutr,* 28:85, 1975.

14. Marktl, W., and Rudas, B.: Screening for risks of cardiovascular disease in children. A preliminary report. *Br J Nutr,* 35:223, 1976.

15. Friedman, G., and Goldberg, S. J.: Concurrent and subsequent serum cholesterols of breast- and formula-fed infants. *Am J Clin Nutr,* 28:42, 1975.

16. Reiser, R.: Saturated fat in the diet and serum cholesterol concentrations: a critical examination of the literature. *Am J Clin Nutr,* 26:524, 1973.

17. Mann, G. V., and Sperry, A.: Studies of a surfactant and cholesteremia in the Maasai. *Am J Clin Nutr,* 27:464, 1974.

18. Dyerberg, J., Bang, H. O., and Hjorne, N.: Fatty acid composition of

the plasma lipids in Greenland Eskimos. *Am J Clin Nutr, 28*:958, 1975.

19. Nichols, A. B., Ravenscroft, C., Lamphiear, D. E., and Ostrander, L. D.: Daily nutritional intake and serum lipid levels. The Tecumseh Study. *Am J Clin Nutr, 29*:1384, 1976.
20. Anderson, J. T., Grande, F., and Keys, A.: Independence of the effects of cholesterol and degree of saturation of the fat in the diet on serum cholesterol in man. *Am J Clin Nutr, 29*:1784, 1976.
21. Jenkins, D. J. A., Leeds, A. R., Newton, C., and Cummings, J. H.: Effects of pectin, guar gum, and wheat fiber on serum cholesterol. *Lancet, 1*:1116, 1975.
22. Potter, J. M. and Nestel, P.: The effects of dietary fatty acids and cholesterol on the milk lipids of lactating mothers and the plasma cholesterol of breast-fed infants. *Am J Clin Nutr, 29*:54, 1976.
23. Witting, L.: Vitamin E–polyunsaturated lipid relationship in diet and tissues. *Am J Clin Nutr, 27*:952, 1974.
24. Pearce, M. L., and Dayton, S.: Incidence of cancer in men on a diet high in polyunsaturated fat. *Lancet, 1*:464, 1971.
25. Mukai, F. H. and Goldstein, B. D.: Mutagenicity of malonaldehyde, a decomposition product of peroxidized polyunsaturated fatty acids. *Science, 191*:868, 1976.
26. Rhoads, G. G., Gulbrandsen, C. L., and Kagan, A.: Serum lipoproteins and coronary heart disease in a population study of Hawaii Japanese men. *N Engl J Med, 294*:293, 1976.
27. Friedman, R. J., Moore, S., and Singal, D. P.: Regression of injury-induced atheromatous lesions in rabbits. *Arch Pathol Lab Med, 100*:189, 1976.
28. Hill, M. J.: Steroid nuclear dehydrogenation and colon cancer. *Am J Clin Nutr, 27*:1475, 1974.
29. Hill, M. J., Drasar, B. S., Williams, R. E. O., Meade, T. W., Cox, A. G., Simpson, J. E. P., and Morson, B. C.: Faecal bile acids and clostridia in patients with cancer of the large bowel. *Lancet, 1*:535, 1975.
30. Monsen, E. R. and Adriaenesens, W.: Fatty acid composition and total lipid of cream and cream substitutes. *Am J Clin Nutr, 22*:458, 1969.
31. Mattson, F. H., Hollenbach, E. J., and Kligman, A. M.: Effect of hydrogenated fat on the plasma cholesterol and triglyceride levels of man. *Am J Clin Nutr, 28*:726, 1975.
32. Schrock, C. G. and Connor, W. J.: Incorporation of the dietary trans-fatty acid (C18:1) into the serum lipids, the serum lipoproteins, and adipose tissue. *Am J Clin Nutr, 28*:1020, 1975.
33. Shulman, R. S., Bhattacharayya, A. K., Connor, W. E., and Fredrichson, D. S.: β-sitosterolemia and xanthomatosis. *N Engl J Med, 294*:482, 1976.

PART II

INORGANIC MACRONUTRIENTS

PART II

CLINICAL CONSIDERATIONS

SODIUM AND POTASSIUM

T HE TWO MINERAL substances found in largest quantity in body fluids are sodium and potassium. The intake of both may vary widely in normal persons, in whom the kidneys regulate what is kept and what is excreted.

The total body sodium (and chloride) contents have been studied.[1] The total body sodium is influenced by skeletal and bone mass; both of these tissues contain large stores of sodium. However, sodium is largely extracellular and, hence, its status is usually ascertained by measurements of serum levels. Marked changes in serum level are always due to disease; nutritional deficiency does not exist. Some degree of sodium depletion may occur in persons who sweat a great deal while working in very hot environments, and this may cause symptoms, such as weakness and muscle cramps. These are easily ameliorated by taking salt. The development of hyponatremia is never dietary in origin and always indicates a more or less serious disturbance of electrolyte balance caused by some disease, or by its energetic treatment. The intake of sodium chloride is to a great extent voluntary, because salt is added in cooking or at the table. The salt intake in those who do not regulate for medical reasons may range between 4 and 15 grams a day, with no detectable difference in body chemistry or in medical history. Although restricting salt intake is useful in treating hypertension, there is no convincing evidence that an excessive intake of salt, much less a normal intake, *causes* hypertension, or anything else. This conclusion seems valid despite eloquent attempts to prove that essential hypertension is caused by excessive salt intake.[2]

As regards potassium, here, too, derangements of its metabolism are almost always due to some serious disease or to some type of energetic treatment of renal, hepatic, or cardiovascular disease. One condition that is often overlooked in this regard is diarrhea that lasts for more than a day or two; it may cause

43

significant potassium depletion. The body potassium is about 90 percent intracellular, and hence, the well-recognized decrease in total body potassium that occurs with age, especially in women,[3] is a reflection of the loss in total muscle mass that occurs with age. A dietary potassium deficiency probably is unknown, but a deficiency in disease is very much more common than is usually recognized. When depletion of body potassium occurs because of disease or its treatment, it usually does not reveal itself by a decrease in serum potassium level.[5] The potassium deficits encountered in medicine vary greatly in degree. The deficit induced by thiazide treatment in otherwise healthy hypertensive patients is usually small and treatable by dietary means alone, i.e. the ingestion of fruits rich in potassium. Cardiac patients given both digitalis and diuretics should receive potassium as such by mouth. However, if digitalis-induced arrhythmias occur, potassium given by mouth may not be adequate. In diabetic acidosis intravenous potassium may be lifesaving.

Striking degrees of unsuspected potassium deficiency are common in cirrhosis of the liver. There seems to be no way of remedying the disorder.

The interrelations between sodium and potassium metabolism have been the subject of a scholarly review.[6] It shows that, at the moment, most of these data do not seem applicable to clinical practice.

REFERENCES

1. Ellis, K. J., Vaswani, A., Zanzi, I., and Cohn, S. H.: Total body sodium and chlorine in normal adults. *Metabolism, 25*:645, 1976.
2. Wiensier, R. L.: Overview: Salt and the development of essential hypertension. *Prev Med, 5*:7, 1976.
3. Cohn, S. H., Vaswani, A., Zanzi, I., Aloria, J. F., Roginsky, M. S., and Ellis, K. J.: Changes in body chemical composition with age measured by total-body neutron activation. *Metabolism, 25*:85, 1976.
4. Carlmark, B., Kromhout, D., and Reizenstein, P.: Total-body potassium measurements in 230 patients. A study of potassium depletion. *Scand J Lab Clin Invest, 35*:617, 1975.
5. Soler, N. G., Jain, S., James, H., and Paton, A.: Potassium status of patients with cirrhosis. *Gut, 17*:152, 1976.
6. Meneely, G. R. and Battarbee, H. D.: Sodium and potassium. *Nutr Rev, 34*:225, 1976.

MAGNESIUM

Although magnesium is a cofactor in a host of enzymic reactions in plant and animal species, its role in human nutrition remains obscure. The human body contains approximately 25 grams of the metal, a fact that indicates its widespread importance and also why a purely nutritional deficiency of the element is uncommon.[1]

Magnesium is distributed in the human body in much the same manner as potassium; it is mainly an intracellular substance. In the plasma around 35 percent of the magnesium is bound to protein. The cerebrospinal fluid contains almost twice as much magnesium as the blood serum.

Since magnesium is a component of chlorophyll and is also found in animal protein, it is abundant in the diet. Most people take around 300 mg per day.

The loss of magnesium in the urine in diabetic acidosis and in the stool in diarrhea may be very large. Nasogastric drainage may also induce large losses. It is, however, not possible to ascribe any specific symptoms to this deficiency. Cirrhosis of the liver is accompanied by low serum concentrations, as is acute pancreatitis. Apparently tetany can occur as a result of hypomagnesemia, but this is rare.

REFERENCES

1. Wacker, W. E. C. and Vallee, B. L.: Magnesium metabolism. N Engl J Med, 259:431 and 475, 1958.

CALCIUM

Ninety-nine percent of the body calcium is in teeth and bones, and hence, the structural role of calcium has been emphasized. However, the bone pool of calcium is far from static. The bones, especially the trabeculae, are part of a highly dynamic system that involves labile bone and also plasma, extracellular tissue fluid, and intracellular fluid calcium concentrations. Orchestrating this complex system are the vitamin 1,25-dihydroxycholecalciferol and the hormones parathormone and calcitonin. The question arises about why abnormal calcium deposits, as in arteries, do not enter this scheme of calcium balance. The answer may be that except in rare instances these deposits contain no osteoblasts or osteoclasts—the bone cells that regulate the amount of calcium in bones.

In the bones themselves, calcium deposition is controlled by more than simple metabolic balances. For example, the degree to which an extremity is used is a factor that determines the calcium content of the bones. Not only are the right-hand bones likely to be larger in a right-handed person, they are likely to be more dense as well.

The normal serum calcium level in man is in the neighborhood of 10 mg per 100 ml (5 meq per liter). Approximately 40 percent of this is bound to serum protein and, hence, un-ionized and presumably physiologically inert. (It still participates in calcium metabolism as a transport form.) The serum calcium level falls when the serum albumin concentration is lowered, but in such cases there is no change in ionizable calcium concentration and no symptoms. A decrease in ionizable calcium level causes tetany as well as a lowering of sensory thresholds.

The recommended dietary allowance of 800 mg per day for "most healthy people" should not be accepted as definitive. Vitamin D regulates calcium absorption from the gut, but there are other phenomena inherent in dietary factors that also influence it. Accordingly, in some parts of the world with diets different from ours, the recommended dietary intakes are lower—in some areas, 50 percent lower. The dietary factors that decrease calcium absorption are incompletely known. For example, although oxalate salts of calcium must form when foods that contain oxalate are taken (see page 176), there is no evidence of any calcium deficiency caused by diets high in oxalate-rich rhubarb, spinach, or certain other leafy vegetables. Similarly, the phytic acid present in grains but ordinarily destroyed by phytase during the leavening of the bread combines with calcium to form insoluble salts. Unleavened bread contains large amounts of phytate, and hence, when this bread is a main part of the diet, impairment of calcium absorption might be expected to be common. Nevertheless, although zinc and iron deficiency may develop in those who eat this bread (see page 71), there is nothing to indicate that any significant amount of calcium deficiency occurs also.

On the other hand, conditions in which steatorrhea occurs are commonly accompanied by hypocalcemia. This is presumed to be due to defective absorption of dietary calcium that results from the combination of the calcium with the excessive fat in the intestines, the combination being insoluble calcium soaps. However, a subnormal absorption of vitamin D in malabsorption syndromes must not be ruled out as a possible factor. Whatever the mechanism, the hypocalcemia may be a significant part of the syndrome.

The ratio between dietary phosphate and calcium content must affect the absorption of the calcium. The usual recommendation is that the ratio be 1.0. However, the American diet at present contains relatively less phosphate so that the Ca/P ratio is greater—sometimes as high as 2.0. The contention that this is unhealthy as regards calcium absorption is supported neither by definitive laboratory data nor by clinical observation. This is not to say that there is no optimal dietary calcium/phosphate ratio, or range of ratios. The fact is simply that there is no way to establish this ratio in man. Despite the fact that available studies seem to indicate that distortion of the Ca/P ratio has no deleterious effects, the fact remains that under certain conditions it may. For example, giving patients with fractures 1 or 2 extra grams of phosphorus, or phosphate, daily has been reported to hasten calcium deposition and bone healing.[1] On the other hand, greatly excessive intakes of phosphate may be harmful (see page 52).

The situation with regard to the effects of dietary protein intake on calcium metabolism is equally unsettled. Whereas earlier workers, i.e. ten to thirty years ago, reported improved calcium balances with protein,[2] recent studies show that a high protein intake leads to calcium loss, chiefly in the urine.[2, 3, 4] An exception appears to occur in adolescent boys, where increased protein was found to improve calcium balance.[5] Perhaps the effect of protein varies with whether the person is or is not in a period of rapid growth. Another exception is perhaps to be found in the effects of soybean protein. In persons who take soybean diets, calcium retention seems to vary with the protein content of what is eaten.[6] At any rate, the mechanism of the calcium loss that may occur in adult men taking very large amounts of protein is not known. The calcium loss caused by a high protein intake has been suggested as the cause of the osteoporosis of the elderly, but this proposition is not supported by clinical observation, for the elderly do not as a rule take high protein diets.

Of all the dietary factors studied in relation to enhancing the absorption of calcium from the gut, only lactose stands out. This effect is, of course, absent in persons with milk tolerance.

The dietary need for calcium is increased in pregnancy, as is commonly recognized, and in lactation, as is often ignored.

In women the total body calcium has been found to fall at a rate of 0.4 percent before age fifty and 1 percent a year thereafter.[7] In men the losses were found to be smaller. (These losses were corrected for weight loss in the elderly.) In women the peak of bone density is around the ages of thirty-five to forty-five, although 10 to 15 percent of apparently normal women show a low bone density as early as the age of twenty-five years. In men bone density is at its peak at age forty-five to fifty-five. At all ages men have much more calcium in them than women, even after allowances are made for differences in weight.[8] However, black women have much more calcium in their bones than white women and even some white men of corresponding age.[9, 10]

The cause of the calcium loss associated with aging is not clear. One factor may be inactivity; it certainly is a factor in the ill, infirm, or immobile.[11] The greater losses in women may be accelerated to some extent by pregnancies and lactation. However, hormonal effects are evidently also important, for the loss of estrogen after the menopause clearly plays a role.[12] Nevertheless, recent studies have shown that when elderly persons who take decreasing amounts of dietary calcium owing to social factors are made to increase their intake, their loss stops and, in fact, over a period of a year or two, may be reversed.[13]

Disease may produce demineralization of bone. Thus, alcoholics have been found to have decreased bone mass.[14]

A factor that still remains to be worked out is the effect of stress. Both physical and strong mental stress create a catabolic state of varying severity in different people. Calcium is lost as part of the catabolic reaction, and there is no indication that this loss can be prevented or reversed by dietary manipulation. However, after the stressful episode is over, the restoration of losses should be attempted.

RECOMMENDATIONS

An intake of 1,000 mg per day should be maintained during life except during periods of immobilization, when administered calcium cannot be retained.

During pregnancy and lactation, an increase of 30 to 50 percent is in order. Increases are also desirable in alcoholic patients and in patients taking anticonvulsant drugs.

REFERENCES

1. Goldsmith, R. S., Woodhouse, C. F., Ingbar, S. H., and Segal, D.: Effect of phosphate supplements in patients with fractures. *Lancet,* *1*:687, 1967.
2. Margen, S., Chu, J.-Y., Kaufmann, N. A., and Calloway, D. H.: Studies in calcium metabolism. I. The calciuretic effect of dietary protein. *Am J Clin Nutr,* 27:584, 1974.
3. Johnson, N. F., Alcantara, E. N., and Linkswiler, H.: Effect of level of protein intake on urinary and fecal calcium and calcium retention of young adult males. *J Nutr,* 100:1425, 1970.
4. Walker, R. M., and Linkswiler, H.: Calcium excretion in the adult male as affected by protein intake. *J Nutr,* 102:1297, 1972.

5. Schwartz, R., Woodcock, N. A., Blakely, J. D., and MacKellar, J.: Metabolic responses of adolescent boys to two levels of dietary magnesium and protein. II. Effect of magnesium and protein level on calcium balance. *Am J Clin Nutr, 26*:519, 1973.

6. Adolph, W. H. and Chen, S.-C.: The utilization of calcium in soybean diets. *J Nutr, 5*:379, 1932.

7. Cohn, S. H., Vaswani, A., Zanzi, I., Aloia, J. F., Roginsky, M. S., and Elbs, K. S.: Changes in body chemical composition with age measured by total-body neutron activation. *Metabolism, 25*:85, 1976.

8. Hopsu, V. K., Kajanoja, P., Telkka, A., and Virtama, D.: The density of small bones of the human extremities with special reference to the reliability of volume measurements. *Anat Ann, 109*:248, 1961.

9. Trotter, M., Broman, G. E., and Peterson, R. H.: Densities of white and Negro skeletons. *J Bone Joint Surg, 42A*:50, 1960.

10. Cohn, S. H., Abesamis, C., Yasamura, S., Aloia, J. F., Zanzi, I., and Ellis, K. J.: Comparative skeletal mass and radial bone mineral content in black and white women. *Metabolism, 26*:171, 1977.

11. Ede, M. C. M. and Burr, R. G.: Circadian rhythm of urinary calcium excretion during immobilization. *Aerosp Med, 44*:495, 1973.

12. Meema, S., Bunker, M. L., and Meema, H. E.: Preventive effect of estrogen on postmenopausal bone loss. *Arch Intern Med, 135*:1436, 1975.

13. Albanese, A. A., Edelson, A. H., Lorenze, E. J., Jr., Woodhull, M. L., and Wein, E. N.: Problems of bone health in the elderly. Ten-year study. *NY State J Med, 75*:326, 1975.

14. Nilsson, E. and Westlin, N. E.: Changes in bone mass in alcoholics. *Clin Orthop, 90*:229, 1973.

PHOSPHATE

Approximately 80 percent of the phosphorus in the body is in bone and teeth. Accordingly, phosphate and calcium metabolism often go together. However, much of the remaining 20 percent of the phosphate exists in small carbohydrate constituents that form during the intermediary metabolism chiefly of carbohydrate and fat. The presence of phosphorus in a variety of lipid compounds constitutes another important function of that element. Hence, it is misleading to assume that the nutritional aspects of calcium and phosphorus must be discussed only in relation to each other. Although it is true that the decline with age of total body calcium and total body phosphorus runs parallel,[1] concentrations of calcium and phosphate are not necessarily parallel in blood serum and among tissues.

In this country the dietary intake of calcium usually exceeds that of phosphorus (although the recommended dietary intake of both is the same). There are regularly striking decreases in serum inorganic phosphate when carbohydrate is eaten or taken by vein.[2] Whether this lasts long enough after an ordinary meal to be physiologically significant is doubtful, but prolonged administration of glucose by vein is certainly harmful. Although the serum inorganic phosphate level falls after intravenous administration of certain peptides,[3] there is no evidence that an ordinary meat meal has this effect. Stress, perhaps, also lowers serum inorganic phosphate level if we are to judge from this effect of epinephrine administration.[3] Adrenal corticoids, which may also be released during stress, exaggerate the fall caused by glucose.[4] In studies made under clinical conditions, the fall in plasma inorganic phosphate concentration during intravenous alimentation was so marked and prolonged as to produce a fall in erythrocyte 2,3-diphosphoglycerate (DPG), and this gives rise to a potentially dangerous high affinity state of the red blood cell hemoglobin. The patients' blood in such cases takes up oxygen in the lungs

51

readily but cannot give it up in the peripheral tissues. A state of tissue hypoxia accordingly develops. In addition to the fall in the erythrocyte 2,3-DPG level, there is also a decrease in adenosine triphosphate (ATP) concentration. This change in ATP concentration may shorten the life of circulating erythrocytes.

As noted before, giving increased amounts of phosphate may, in some circumstances, increase the deposition of calcium in bone. However, it may stimulate the parathyroid glands. Although adding 1.0 gram of phosphate to the normal intake in patients with osteoporosis has no such effect,[5] larger amounts in normal persons do have this adverse effect.[6]

RECOMMENDATIONS

In normal persons the intake of phosphorous should be around 1.0 gram per day.

REFERENCES

1. Cohn, S. H., Vaswami, A., Zanzi, I., Alvia, J. F., Roginsky, M. S., and Ellis, K. J.: Changes in body chemical composition with age measured by total-body neutron activation. *Metabolism*, 25:85, 1976.
2. Henneman, D. H., Altschule, M. D., and Goncz, R. M.: Carbohydrate metabolism in brain disease. II. Glucose metabolism in schizophrenic, manic-depressive, and involutional psychoses. *Arch Intern Med*, 94:402, 1954.
3. Henneman, D. H., Altschule, M. D., and Goncz, R. M.: Effect of intravenous administration of glutathione in man on blood glucose, some other blood carbohydrates, and serum inorganic phosphate. *Metabolism*, 4:433, 1955.
4. Henneman, D. H., Altschule, M. D., and Goncz, R. M.: Carbohydrate metabolism in brain disease. IV. Effect of hydrocortisone and corticotropin (ACTH) on the metabolic effects of administered glucose in patients with chronic schizophrenic and manic-depressive psychoses. *Arch Intern Med*, 95:241, 1955.
5. Goldsmith, R. S., Jowsey, J., Dubé, W. J., Riggs, B. L., Arnaud, C. D., and Kelly, P. J.: Effects of phosphorus supplementation on serum parathyroid hormone and bone morphology in osteoporosis. *J Clin Endocrinol Metab*, 43:523, 1976.
6. Bell, R. R., Draper, H. H., Tzeng, D. Y. M., Shin, H. K., and Schmidt, C. R.: Physiological responses of adults to foods containing phosphate additives. *J Nutr*, 107:42, 1977.

PART III

TRACE ELEMENTS

IRON

Iron is present in the human body in amounts and concentrations too large to justify designating it a nutritional trace element. It is present in amounts of 3 to 5 grams in the adult human body. On the other hand, owing to certain peculiarities in the metabolism of iron, the daily metabolic requirement (not the amount that must be taken in the diet) is only a milligram or two. Absorption of the ingested iron is poor, and hence, the daily dietary requirement is approximately ten times what is absorbed into the bloodstream.

Iron is involved in many different types of metabolic activity. Perhaps its best-known action is as the metallic component of blood hemoglobin in its function of oxygen delivery to the tissues. More than half of the iron in the body is in the blood hemoglobin. Another one-third exists in storage forms, i.e. ferritin and hemosiderin. Ferritin is the main storage form of iron in the liver and the reticuloendothelial system. It has a high molecular weight and is composed of a protein shell (apoferritin) synthesized by the liver and surrounding a core of ferric hydroxide. The more commonly known hemosiderin is probably a complex aggregate of partially denatured ferritin molecules.

The remainder of the body iron is scattered as parts of a wide variety of important tissue enzymes. In some of these, e.g. peroxidase, the status of the iron is similar to that of the iron in hemoglobin, that is, in association with porphyrin moieties. In other enzymes the relation of the iron to the rest of the molecule is different. In hemoglobin the iron must exist with a valence of two; oxidation to a valence of three forms methemoglobin, which does not transport oxygen, and there is evidence that trivalent iron in the diet is less satisfactory than the divalent. Less is known about the iron in the tissue enzymes.

The seeming paradox of 3 to 5 grams of iron in the body and the daily requirement of less than one thousandth of that amount requires explanation. Most of the iron in the body is reused again and again. Six hundred and fifty grams of hemoglobin are present in the circulating red blood cells, and since approximately 1 percent of these cells die every day, the hemoglobin in them, i.e. approximately 6.5 grams, is broken down by the reticulo-endothelial cells of the spleen and liver. The iron in this hemo-globin enters the blood plasma where it is bound to the plasma protein called transferrin, or siderophilin, to be carried to wher-ever needed. At least part of this iron is introduced into proto-porphyrin in the bone marrow, making thereby the heme portion of hemoglobin. The latter is taken into the newly-born red blood cells in the bone marrow. This seemingly perfect system has a serious flaw: There is no mechanism for regulating losses of iron from the body. These losses may be in the form of a visible loss of blood such as menstrual flow, bleeding hemorrhoids, etc. However, there may be invisible losses of blood. The stool normally contains less than 1 milliliter of blood per day, but in persons taking salicylates this loss is usually ten times as much, although still invisible. Larger amounts may be lost in the stool in hookworm disease. In addition, there is loss of iron as such. For example, in pregnancy some of the mother's iron is given to the fetus. A nursing mother gives her three-month-old infant approximately 0.5 mg of iron a day in her milk. This is 25 to 50 percent of what she absorbs from her food.[1] In all persons some iron is lost in the sweat and a large amount in the dead skin cells that flake off all day. In some conditions of stress the urinary excretion of hydroxybenzoic acids increases, and these chelate iron (and other metals), removing them from the body.[2] One hydroxybenzoic acid is salicylic acid, and those who take large amounts of it will lose iron in the urine thereby. There is no way in which the body can regulate or prevent the loss of iron, and hence, unless this loss is compensated for by suitably increased intakes, iron depletion must result. Failure to increase the dietary intake of iron in these circumstances is common, and iron defici-ency is by far the most common nutritional deficiency in all parts of the world, especially in women.[3] However, in one population study anemia was also common in men.[4] The incidence of anemia in children of both sexes was notable.[4] In the cases of the children and many of the adult women, the intake of dietary iron was low.

There is no good regulatory mechanism to insure that the right amount of iron gets into the body. There is, moreover, no complete understanding of the mechanisms that have been found to act in iron absorption. For example, after the loss of blood has produced a need for more iron, the percent of ingested iron absorbed from the intestinal contents increases, but the mechanism of this phenomenon is not known. At first glance the phenomenon would appear to be solely a response to an increased need for iron, but the best evidence indicates that the phenomenon is also owing to increased erythropoiesis. If no increase in erythropoiesis occurs after a hemorrhage, there is no evidence of increased iron absorption from the gut. In anemic persons in whom erythropoiesis is not increased, i.e. in the anemias of infection, uremia, neoplasia, or chronic trauma, the absorption of iron is not increased, but in such cases the iron stores in the tissues may be normal. Thus in all these anemias and in posthemorrhagic anemia, the serum iron level is low, but only in the last is iron absorption increased and only in the last is erythropoiesis (normally) increased. Some authors have assumed that the low serum iron level that characterizes the aforementioned conditions in which erythropoiesis is depressed is related to the fact that the greatest part of the serum iron is there because of red blood cell breakdown. If, for example, the red blood cell count is half normal, the number of cells dying each day will be half the normal and so their contribution to the circulating iron pool must be half normal. However convincing this explanation might appear to be, its validity is greatly impaired by the findings in the anemia of vitamin B_6 deficiency. In this condition, despite the marked decrease in erythropoiesis and the consequent decrease of the number (not the precentage) of red blood cells that die each day, the serum iron level is extremely high.

It is clear from all this that the mechanism of iron absorption from the intestinal contents is not known. Attempts to understand how this process is regulated have likewise been unfruitful. In this connection, it is important to note that if very large amounts of iron are taken by mouth, an abnormal amount is absorbed from the intestinal contents. Some of the excess iron so absorbed is deposited in the various parts of the body and may be highly damaging. However, the storage of the iron so deposited differs somewhat from that observed in idiopathic hemochromatosis.[5] The anemia of infection might offer a clue as to what occurs if appropriate studies were made. In this condition, the serum iron level is very low: It may be less than half the normal. The serum iron-binding protein—the transferrin-concentration—remains close to normal. Giving iron by mouth does not increase the serum iron level or alleviate the anemia. These findings have led to the conclusion that infection in some way prevents the absorption of iron from the gut. This may well be true, but it has also been shown that in infection the liver may accumulate large stores of iron. This apparent diversion of iron from the plasma (and the bone marrow) has never been explained. Diversion of a metal from the plasma to the liver in persons with infection has also been observed with zinc (see page 71). In infections other than hepatitis, the serum zinc level falls and large amounts of that metal move into the liver.

Despite the conservation of iron in the body, manifested by the persistent recycling of the iron from overaged red blood cells, the total absence of regulation of iron loss and the seemingly haphazard regulation of intake make it difficult to maintain a good balance on any day. The presence of storage iron makes up deficits in intake or compensates for losses up to a point. However, these stores amount to only 1.0 or 1.5 grams out of the total iron and are easily exhausted when there are constant or repeated losses that are not made up by increased intakes. A state of severe iron deficiency can also occur without serious evident losses in growing children whose supply at birth or in infancy is inadequate.

One of the distressing features of iron metabolism in man is that it is not easily studied. Although the serum iron level may be used empirically to help diagnose the type of anemia present, it affords no information about the amount of the iron stores. Actually, the need for a method to estimate iron stores is very great. A mild deficiency of bodily iron may not be revealed by hemoglobin or hematocrit readings. Measurement of the serum transferrin saturation (about 32% is normal) will detect twice as many patients with developing iron deficiency anemia as do the hemoglobin and hematocrit measurements. The same is true of the red blood cell protoporphyrin content, but this measurement is not widely used. In any case, none of these measurements can show changes until the iron stores are completely exhausted. Accordingly, a method is needed for the detection of changes in the amount of stored iron when this value is changing up or down remote from the point of total exhaustion. Such a measurement now seems to exist. The measurement of serum ferritin concentration has recently been suggested as a means of ascertaining the magnitude of the iron stores of the body.[6, 7, 8] This new test is believed by some not only to permit the accurate evaluation of the body's iron stores but also to show the effects of iron ingestion as such and of changes in the diet, including fortification. One study in which this method was used has already been published.[9] In anemic patients with no evidence of chronic inflammatory or hepatic disease, the values are very low. In patients with hemochromatosis or patients who had received twenty or more transfusions, the values are fifty to two hundred times the normal! In patients with chronic inflammatory states, the serum ferritin level is as much as fifteen times the normal, despite the fact that some are anemic. Patients with anemia associated with chronic liver disease show similar findings. For a given amount of stainable iron seen in bone marrow aspirates, the patients with the chronic disorders show much higher serum ferritin values than patients with simple iron deficiency. Patients with macrocytic anemias and hemolytic anemias are found to have high serum ferritin values. The test appears to distinguish uncomplicated iron deficiency states from uncomplicated anemias associated with chronic diseases. This is an important finding because the latter anemias do not respond to iron,[10] and giving iron to them, or to others who do not need it, will probably produce overload.[11] Although more recent studies show that the serum ferritin level does not always rise when the iron stores increase above normal,[12, 13] the test still distinguishes iron deficiency anemia from the anemia of chronic diseases such as infection and neoplasm. Here we have another example of biochemical measurement, originally hailed as a means of improving understanding of disease processes, that turns out to be itself inexplicable but remains a useful test under clinical conditions.

On the whole, however, physicians will still have to make clinical conclusions based on their evaluations of the situation in each particular patient. The symptoms of iron deficiency are not specific. They include lassitude and fatigability, mental irritability or depression, exercise-induced tachycardia, chilly or cold feelings on exposure, and a tendency to retain fluid in the tissues. Children show a failure to grow and thrive. Only in extreme cases does shortness of breath on exertion occur. This is true because changes in red blood cell chemistry (an increase in red blood cell 2,3-diphosphoglycerate) facilitate the offloading of oxygen in the tissues, compensating for much of the lack of oxygen-carrying capacity caused by a low hemoglobin concentration. There is evidence of decreased bacteriocidal effectiveness of the leukocytes in iron deficiency states,[14, 15] and clinically, there is a high correlation between iron deficiency and a variety of infections.

A physician who finds a low hemoglobin or hematocrit value in a patient will naturally think of iron deficiency anemia. However, he will have to seek confirmation in the patient's history. In the first place, one third of menstruating women have no iron reserves detectable on staining the bone marrow.[16] As regards iron intake, a history of low intake of meat, including liver and kidneys, or of fish should arouse suspicion. The other good natural source of food iron is green vegetables, but many find them too expensive out of season or not very appetizing frozen or canned. Moreover, throwing away the cooking water destroys much of the value of green vegetables as a source of iron. On the other hand, in some areas the drinking water, or beverages prepared from it, may contain large amounts of iron, either naturally or as a result of being carried through iron pipes. In addition, using crude iron vessels in cooking may cause a very large increase in the intake of iron.

Certain factors affect the absorption of iron. Ascorbic acid, taken either as such or in food, enhances it. However, no matter how rich a diet may be in iron, the absorption of the food iron is reduced by some factors. One may be the taking of a diet consisting entirely of cow's milk, as in infancy. Studies show that the absorption of dietary iron is greatly reduced by the ingestion of calcium and phosphate together (as in milk), whereas giving either calcium or phosphate alone has little effect.[17] In some cases, however, there is evidence that the impaired absorption of iron is due to a type of hypersensitivity to cow's milk that injures the lining of the intestinal tract.[18] Another cause of defective absorption of food iron is the use of unleavened Middle East bread.[19] This contains a considerable amount of phytate, a vegetable substance that chelates iron and prevents its absorption. (The same is true of zinc—see page 71). Another wheat product, bran, is rich in iron, but the cellulose in it chelates the metal and reduces its absorption so much when it is fed in a dose of 36 gm per day that it lowers the serum iron level.[20] In addition, there are a number of medications, some of them commonly used, that inhibit iron absorption.[21] These are antacids that contain magnesium trisilicate (including Tums®), neomycin, allopurinal (used to treat gout and other conditions of hyperuricemia), and cholestyramine (used to lower serum cholesterol level). As has been pointed out, there may be excessive losses of iron in the stool and urine when aspirin or other salicylates are taken. A major cause of failure to absorb iron is removal of part of the stomach, perhaps with closing off of the duodenum.[22] To complicate matters, iron deficiency itself impairs the absorption of iron from the intestine.[23, 24]

The history relative to the state of iron nutrition must also go into the matter of blood loss, menstrual or pathological.

If the amount of iron taken in or retained is low, iron must be given as such. How much? This question cannot be answered in any definite way. The physician must base his conclusion on experience. He must use restoration of the hemoglobin and hematocrit readings to normal if they are low, and maintenance of normal level if they are found. The validity of these criteria is weakened by a well-known clinical phenomenon: When iron is given to persons with iron-deficiency anemia, they feel markedly better days before the blood hemoglobin and hematocrit values rise measurably. This phenomenon lends support to Beutler's opinion that many of the symptoms of iron deficiency are due, at least at rest, to impairment of the actions of a variety of tissue enzymes and not to a lack of blood hemoglobin.

With iron-deficiency anemia as widespread as it is, there have naturally been attempts to prevent or eradicate it by putting iron into what many people eat, especially cereals, breads, and bread products. This effort has been accepted as not only laudable but successful by several categories of people, including some nutritionists, who deal with masses of people and not, like physicians, with individuals. However, the most enthusiastic supporters of these efforts are to be found in the advertising industry. The wish is clearly father to the thought, but the thought is not acceptable without scrutiny. The recent literature contains a study that deserves every praise for the enormous effort and careful planning involved, and the careful conclusions developed.[25] In this study, carried out in a clinic that has consistently produced outstanding work, the first preparations involved making radioactively tagged iron compounds and growing corn and wheat in soil enriched with these tagged isotopes. Another preparation involved giving tagged ferric citrate intravenously to a calf, which was later used as a source for radioactively tagged iron-containing heme in its meat. The tagged grains and tagged meat were then fed. It was found that the absorptions of inorganic ferrous sulphate and ferric chloride were equal and were the same as the absorption of the tagged iron in the grains. These absorptions were, however, disappointingly low, averaging about 3 percent of the amount ingested. However, when the inorganic-tagged ferric chloride was given together with meat, 27 percent of it was absorbed. The feeding of radioactively tagged heme as hamburger steak was followed by the absorption of 20 percent of the tagged iron in it. Evidently there is something in meat that enhances, or something in grain that decreases, the absorption of iron salts, both ferrous sulfate and ferric chloride. The authors concluded that iron fortification was not useful when the meal comprised chiefly vegetables. Another excellent study by the same group confirms and extends these observations.[16] In addition, it has been shown that infants, like adults, absorb iron poorly from fortified cereals.[26] These studies, too, showed that meat and fish enhance the absorption of dietary iron, whereas another source of animal protein, eggs, does not. (Of course, eggs contain iron of their own.) The role of animal proteins in the absorption of nonheme iron is still being studied.[27] The great effect of animal protein in enhancing the absorption of iron was confirmed, as was the lesser effect of egg protein.

Two other studies by other workers led in the same direc-

of serum ferritin as an index of iron stones. *N Engl J Med, 290*: 1213, 1974.

10. Cartwright, G. E. and Lee, G. R.: The anemia of chronic disorders. *Br J Haematol, 21*:147, 1971.

11. Crosby, W. H.: Iron enrichment. One's food, another's poison. *Arch Intern Med, 126*:911, 1970.

12. Wands, J. R., Rowe, J. A., Mezey, S. F., Waterbury, L. A., Wright, J. R., Halliday, J. W., Isselbacher, K. J., and Powell, L. W.: Normal serum ferritin concentrations in precirrhotic hemochromatosis. *N Engl J Med, 294*:302, 1976.

13. Crosby, W. H.: Serum ferritin fails to indicate hemochromatosis—nothing gold can stay. *N Engl J Med, 294*:333, 1976.

14. Chandra, R. K.: Reduced bactericidal capacity of polymorphs in iron deficiency. *Arch Dis Child, 48*:864, 1973.

15. Sharra, A. J., Selvaraj, R. J., Paul, B. B., Straus, R. R., Jacobs, A. A., and Mitchell, G. W., Jr.: Bactericidal activities of phagocytes in health and disease. *Am J Clin Nutr, 27*:629, 1974.

16. Cook, J. D. and Monsen, E. R.: Food absorption. Use of a semi-synthetic diet to study the absorption of non-heme iron. *J Clin Nutr, 28*:1289, 1975.

17. Monsen, E. R. and Cook, J. D.: Food iron absorption in human subjects. IV. The effects of calcium and phosphate salts on the absorption of non-heme iron. *Am J Clin Nutr, 29*:1142, 1976.

18. Woodruff, C. W., and Clark, J. L.: The role of fresh cow's milk in iron deficiency. I. Albumin turnover in infants with iron-deficiency anemia. *Am J Dis Child, 124*:18, 1972.

19. Mahloudji, M., Reinhold, J. G., Hagshenass, M., Ronaghy, H. R., Spivey Fox, M. R., and Halstead, J. A.: Combined zinc and iron compared with iron supplementation of diets of 6- to 12-year-old village school children in southern Iran. *Am J Clin Nutr, 28*:121, 1975.

20. Jenkins, D. J. A., Hill, M. S., and Cummings, J. H.: Effects of wheat fiber on blood lipids, fecal steroid excretion and serum iron. *Am J Clin Nutr, 28*:1408, 1975.

21. Gaginella, T. S.: Drug-induced malabsorption. *Drug Therapy.* December, 1975, p. 88.

22. Mahmud, K., Ripley, D., Swaim, W., and Doscherhoumen, A.: Hematologic complications of partial gastrectomy. *Ann Surg, 177*:432, 1973.

23. Kimber, C. and Weintraub, L. R.: Malabsorption of iron secondary to iron deficiency. *N Engl J Med, 279*:453, 1968.

24. Gross, S. J., Stuart, M. J., Swender, P. T., and Oski, F. A.: Malabsorption of iron in children with iron deficiency. *J Pediatr, 88*:795, 1976.

25. Layrisse, M., Marting-Torres, C., Cook, J. D., Walker, R., and Finch, C. A.: Iron fortification of food: its measurement by the extrinsic tag method. *Blood, 41*:333, 1973.
26. Cook, J. D. and Monsen, E. R.: Food iron absorption in human subjects. III. Comparison of the effect of animal proteins on non-heme iron absorption. *Am J Clin Nutr, 29*:859, 1976.
27. Woodruff, C. W., Latham, S., and McDavid, S.: Iron nutrition in breast-fed infants. *J Pediatr, 90*:36, 1977.
28. Amine, E. K. and Hegsted, D. M.: Biological assessment of available iron in food products. *J Agric Food Chem, 22*:470, 1974.
29. Waddell, J.: The bioavailability of iron sources and their utilization in food enrichment. *Fed Proc, 33*:1779, 1974.
30. Layrisse, M., Martinez-Torres, C., Renzi, M., Velez, F., and Gonzalez, M.: Sugar as a vehicle for iron fortification. *Am J Clin Nutr, 29*:8, 1976.
31. Bjorn-Rasmussen, E., Halberg, L., Magnusson, B., Rossander, L., Swanberg, B., and Arvidsson, B.: Measurement of iron absorption from composite meals. *Am J Clin Nutr, 29*:772, 1976.
32. Velez, A., Restrepo, A., Vitale, J. J., and Hellerstein, E. E.: Folic acid deficiency secondary to iron deficiency in man. *Am J Clin Nutr, 19*:27, 1966.
33. Chanarin, I.: Diagnosis of folate deficiency in pregnancy. *Acta Obstet Gynecol Scand 4:Supp.* 7:39, 1967.
34. Hines, E. D., Hoffbrand, A. V., and Mollin, D. L.: The hematological complications following partial gastrectomy. *Am J Med, 43*:555, 1967.
35. Roberts, P. D., St. John, D. J. B., Spinea, R., Stewart, J. S., Baird, I. M., Coghill, N. F., and Morgan, J. O.: Apparent folate deficiency in iron-deficiency anemia. *Br J Haematol, 20*:165, 1971.

COPPER

T HERE IS A WEALTH of material in the biochemical literature on the role of copper. The metal is a constituent of important enzymes and is an essential cofactor in the activity of others. However, this information cannot be related to either health, or its absence, in man.

Copper is recognized as a cause of disease when it accumulates excessively, causing Wilson's disease (hepatolenticular degeneration). In this condition the metal accumulates in many tissues, causing symptoms as a consequence of the large amounts in the brain and liver. This is not a nutritional disease; it is owing to a hereditary lack of ceruloplasmin, the copper-binding protein of the blood. (Approximately 90 percent of the serum copper exists as a part of the ceruloplasmin molecule, and when this is lacking, small amounts of the metal may be loosely bound to plasma albumin.) It should be noted that in Wilson's disease, although tissue copper concentrations are extremely high, the serum concentration is very low.

In all acute stress conditions, in normal pregnancy, and during the taking of oral contraceptives, the serum copper level rises markedly, owing to an increase in plasma ceruloplasmin concentration. The findings in women who take oral contraceptives were recently discussed by Prasad et al.[1] Neither the cause nor the usefulness of this phenomenon is known. At any rate it is clear that the serum copper level does not indicate the tissue copper concentration nor the state of copper nutrition.

Isolated nutritional copper deficiency, although it has been studied extensively in animals, has only rarely been recognized in man. There is a syndrome of copper deficiency in infants which is probably best considered as due to a disorder of copper transport rather than a deficiency of intake.[2] A similar syndrome, also rare, may occur in infants with excessive protein loss via the gut.[3] Severe copper deficiency may also occur in malabsorp-

67

tion syndromes and in patients maintained for long periods on intravenous alimentation.[4, 5] In all these cases, anemia, neutropemia, low serum copper and iron concentrations, and, inexplicably, bone demineralization are found.

Almost half a century ago there was some discussion about the possibility that an iron-resistant anemia in milk-fed infants might be due to copper deficiency—at least it seemed to respond to the administration of copper.[6] Although this situation is not very common, there is still frequent comment as regards the need for copper in iron absorption. However, the extreme rarity of dietary copper inadequacy except when a grossly distorted diet is taken makes this deficiency unimaginable.

Nursing women give their three-month-old infants approximately 3.5 mg of copper a day in milk.[7] What effect this has on the mother's nutrition is not clear, and in any case, if any deficiency did occur in her, it might be masked by the high serum ceruloplasmin level.

RECOMMENDATIONS

There is no need to be concerned about copper deficiency in normal persons.

REFERENCES

1. Prasad, A. S., Oberleas, V., Lei, K. Y., Moghissi, K. S., and Strayker, J. C.: Effect of oral contraceptives in nutrients: 1. Minerals. *Am J Clin Nutr,* 28:577, 1975.
2. Sturgeon, P. and Brubaker, C.: Copper deficiency in infants: a syndrome characterized by hypocupremia, iron deficiency anemia, and hypoproteinemia. *Am J Dis Child,* 92:254, 1956.
3. Wilson, J. F., Lahey, M. E., and Heiner, D. C.: Studies on iron metabolism. V. Further observations on cow's milk-induced gastrointestinal bleeding in infants with iron deficiency anemia. *J Pediatr,* 84:335, 1974.
4. Vilter, R. W., Bozian, R. C., Hess, E. V., Zellner, D. C., and Petering, H. G.: Manifestations of copper deficiency in a patient with systemic sclerosis on intravenous hyperalimentation. *N Engl J Med,* 291:188, 1974.

5. Fleming, C. R., Hodges, R. E., and Hurley, L. S.: A prospective study of serum copper and zinc levels in patients receiving total parenteral nutrition. *Am J Clin Nutr*, 29:70, 1976.

6. Josephs, H.: Treatment of anemia of infancy with iron and copper. *Bull Johns Hopkins Hosp*, 49:246, 1931.

7. Picciano, M. F. and Guthrie, H. A.: Copper, iron, and zinc contents of mature human milk. *Am J Clin Nutr*, 29:242, 1976.

ZINC

Z INC IS IMPORTANT in many biological processes in plants and animals. Some of these functions are fairly well defined, particularly those that relate to its role as the metal in a number of metalloenzymes, such as carbonic anhydrase, alkaline phosphatase, pancreatic carboxypeptidases, and a number of dehydrogenases, including alcohol, lactic, glutamate, glyceraldehyde-3-phosphate, and malate dehydrogenase.[1] Zinc is also important in protein synthesis, being part of, or necessary for, the activity of DNA– and RNA–polymerase.

Nutritional zinc deficiency has been extensively studied in birds and mammals, and a variety of syndromes have been described in these organisms.[2, 3, 4]

Although there is much evidence that zinc deficiency causes disease in many mammalian and avian species, the evidence with regard to man is less abundant. Nevertheless, the evidence is convincing, although to some extent unpredictable in nature. For one thing, although zinc is essential for the working of the enzyme carbonic anhydrase—a substance essential for the removal of carbon dioxide from the tissues to the blood and then from the blood in the lungs to the air—marked depression of carbonic anhydrase activity by certain drugs does not produce respiratory acidosis. (Whatever acidosis occurs when these drugs are taken is due to their markedly depressing effect on renal carbonic anhydrase activity.) We also know that in pernicious anemia, in which patients usually take a diet low in zinc by preference, the zinc or carbonic anhydrase in the red blood cells may be perfectly normal. We know nothing about the effect of zinc deficiencies on the function mediated by the other listed enzymes in producing symptoms in man.

In man, zinc deficiency appears to develop only in the presence of disease or owing to gross distortions of diet (or both), and several disorders in man have been shown to be due to zinc deficiency.[2, 3, 4] However, serum zinc levels do not necessarily afford a good indication of tissue zinc levels. In a variety of febrile illnesses, the urine output of zinc falls markedly, despite which the plasma concentration is also found decreased. In these conditions there is an influx of zinc into the liver (accompanied by a similar influx of amino acids into that organ). The zinc thus trapped in the liver seems to be bound, and hence probably physiologically inert.[5] On the other hand, in the presence of liver damage, as in viral hepatitis, there is a fall in plasma zinc level and an increase in urine zinc output.[6] In still another condition, the postoperative state, zinc excretion also increases.[7, 8] The mechanism of this loss is unknown, since if anything, zinc accumulates in wounds. Is the loss part of the catabolic state of trauma, or is it due to immobility, or both? We do not know. At any rate, it is evident that without data of additional studies, the serum zinc level cannot be used diagnostically. Accordingly, the finding of low serum zinc levels in apparently normal American children and infants[9] cannot be interpreted clinically.

The malabsorption syndromes may produce zinc deficiency, not an unexpected finding. Similarly, hemodialysis may also produce zinc deficiency and give rise to a need for supplementation. There is no indication that psychiatric stress affects zinc nutrition, although it is known that the brains of some chronic schizophrenic patients show abnormally low concentrations of zinc in the hippocampus.[10] Zinc deficiency owing to distorted diet may have several mechanisms. In the Middle East the unleavened bread commonly used contains a great excess of phytate, a nonabsorbable vegetable substance, that binds zinc (as well as other metals). Some males who eat a large amount of this bread develop a typical syndrome, hypogonadal dwarfism, owing to a deficient release of gonadotropin. It may be ameliorated if zinc is taken by mouth.[11] The same disease has also been reported in a few girls.[12] It may be more common than that but difficult to recognize because many girls are small anyway, and in any case gonadal insufficiency owing to other causes may overshadow this syndrome. The availability of zinc in wheat is increased by leavening.

In the Western world, some degree of zinc deficiency, usually not recognized, is common because of the reliance on processed cereals. Zinc is plentiful in whole grain cereals as well as in animal protein. Customary methods of processing the cereals result in the loss of approximately 80 percent of the contained zinc.[13] This is not replaced, unlike part of the iron simultaneously removed. In some underdeveloped regions, the large intake of certain plant proteins (soy and other) may also prevent the absorption of normal amounts of zinc. Nursing mothers give their three-month-old infants approximately 3.5 mg of zinc daily in the milk.[14] Whether this has any significant effect on the mothers' zinc nutrition is not known. Evidently this amount of zinc is adequate for the infant, as indicated by measurements of blood carbonic anhydrase activity. This activity, very low at birth, increases rapidly early in life.[15]

Moderate degrees of zinc deficiency in man may cause their effects through a number of mechanisms. One clearly is vitamin A deficiency.[16] Low serum zinc levels are associated with the inability to mobilize the liver stores of vitamin A. This may be due to a deficiency of a retinol-binding plasma protein. The vitamin deficiency may be cured by giving zinc.[17]

This regulatory effect of zinc on the utilization of vitamin A in man may account for the effect of zinc on wound healing discussed by a number of authors as summarized by Henkin.[18] It is known that vitamin A is required for the synthesis of collagen in scar tissue (page 90). However, the role of zinc in protein synthesis may provide an alternative explanation for its effect in accelerating wound healing. Whatever the mechanisms of this clinical effect may be, the poor wound healing due to zinc deficiency is very important, for it must be common in the Western world—and perhaps in other areas—in which distorted diets give dietary zinc deficiency to persons otherwise healthy. Of course, patients who have low serum zinc levels associated with diseases mentioned earlier also exhibit poor wound healing. Although this effect of zinc has been worked out only in traumatic wounds, it may also apply to other types of tissue damage. It is worthy of note that the plasma zinc level falls in patients with myocardial infarction.[19]

Still another factor must be considered. The metal cadmium interferes with the action of zinc at the cellular level. The increasing importance of cadmium as a pollutant in our culture may be playing a role in producing the symptoms of zinc deficiency in persons who may not be deficient in zinc itself.

Patients with alcoholic cirrhosis exhibit low serum zinc concentrations.[20] This situation with respect to alcoholism is complicated in that a deficient zinc intake may be a factor in what occurs. Patients with alcoholic brain disease have very low hippocampal zinc concentrations.[10] However, not only is the mechanism responsible for this cerebral change not established, but the role of the brain zinc deficiency in causing symptoms is not known. Nevertheless, certain facts must not be forgotten. The hippocampus occupies a key position in the limbic system, the complex of structures involved in emotional responses, both behavioral and bodily. The hippocampus is also important in memory processing, in controlling arousal, and for regulating the excitatory states of the higher brain centers. The hippocampus, in addition, influences the pituitary-adrenal system and is sensitive to small changes in circulating hormone concentrations. The functions of the hippocampus appear to be related to the nerve fiber concentrations of zinc.[21] If the zinc deficiency is responsible for abnormal functioning of the limbic system in alcoholics, it does not seem to do so by interfering with the action of neurotransmitters.

Zinc has recently been suggested as a treatment for acne.[22] However, the doses suggested seem too large to be merely repairing a deficiency.

If zinc is regularly removed from our food, why not replace it? This is not easy, because an excessive zinc intake causes copper deficiency.[23] (One of the manifestations of copper deficiency is a rise in serum cholesterol concentration, a fact that has led some authors to fall into the trap of believing that atherosclerosis is caused by copper deficiency brought on by excessive intakes of zinc.)

Although there are some discrepancies (see page 71), for the most part workers in this field agree that female hormonal changes—at least those that occur during pregnancy or during the taking of contraceptive pills—cause a fall in serum zinc level.[25] This fall is, however, accompanied by, or is perhaps the result of, a rise in erythrocyte zinc content. Since pregnancy or the taking of contraceptive pills causes a rise in serum copper level (page 67), the question arises whether the fall in serum zinc concentration should be taken as evidence of a disturbance of the nutritional zinc/copper ratio and hence, an indication for an increase in zinc intake. This seems unlikely in women whose zinc intake is optimal, but since an optimal zinc intake is probably not universal in American women, the question remains open. The best solution is to have the patient take a diet adequate in zinc.

Contrarily, when the serum copper level rises in stress, during pregnancy, or as a result of taking oral contraceptives, does this change represent a shift in the nutritional zinc/copper ratio, and should dietary zinc supplements be given? Again there are no data on which to base a judgment. However, the serum levels of zinc (or copper) do not reliably indicate the nutritional state, and hence, the distorted serum ratio by itself should not be a cause of deep concern. Nevertheless, if the stress involves extensive tissue damage, giving supplemental zinc might be desirable. But how much must be given to remedy acute losses, probably superimposed on chronic deficiency? We do not know. However, experience shows that around 200 mg per day, as the sulphate, is tolerable and does no harm.

RECOMMENDATIONS

A diet rich in zinc comprises meat, seafood, and whole grains. Processed grains have lost most of the metal.

REFERENCES

1. Vallee, B. L.: Zinc biochemistry: a perspective. *Trends in Biochemistry,* 2:88, 1976.
2. Hoekstra, W. G.: Present knowledge of zinc in nutrition. In *Present Knowledge in Nutrition* (3rd ed.). New York, The Nutrition Foundation, 1967, p. 141.
3. Halsted, J. A., Smith, J. C., Jr., and Irwin, M. I.: A conspectus of research on zinc requirements of man. *J Nutr, 104*:347, 1974.
4. Sunderman, F. W., Jr.: Current status of zinc deficiency in the pathogenesis of neurological, dermatological, and musculoskeletal disorders. *Ann Clin Lab Sci, 5*:132, 1975.

5. Wannamacher, R. W., Jr., Dinterman, R. E., Pekarek, R. S., Barelloni, P. J., and Beisel, W. R.: Urinary amino acid excretion during experimentally induced sandfly fever in man. *Am J Clin Nutr, 28*:110, 1975.

6. Henkin, R. I. and Smith, F. R.: Zinc and copper metabolism in acute viral hepatitis. *Am J Med Sci, 264*:401, 1972.

7. Hentzel, J. H., De Weese, M. S., and Pories, W. J.: Significance of magnesium and zinc metabolism in the surgical patient. *Arch Surg, 95*:991, 1967.

8. Kahn, A. M. and Gordon, H. E.: Alterations in zinc metabolism following surgical operations. *Surg Gynecol Obstet, 128*:88, 1969.

9. Hambridge, K. M., Walravens, P. A., Brown, R. M., Webster, J., White, S., Anthony, M., and Roth, M. L.: Zinc nutrition of preschool children in the Denver Head Start program. *Am J Clin Nutr, 29*:734, 1976.

10. McLardy, T.: Hippocampal zinc and structural deficit in brains from chronic alcoholics and some schizophrenics. *J Orthomol Psychiat, 4*:32, 1975.

11. Prasad, A. S., Miale, A., Farid, Z., Sandstead, H. H., and Darby, W. J.: Biochemical studies in dwarfism, hypogonadism and anemia. *AMA Arch Intern Med, 3*:407, 1963.

12. Ronaghy, H. A. and Halsted, J. A.: Zinc deficiency occurring in females. Report of two cases. *Am J Clin Nutr, 28*:831, 1975.

13. Mertz, W.: The effects of zinc in man: nutritional considerations. In W. J. Pories et al. (Eds.): *Clinical Applications of Zinc Metabolism,* Springfield, Ill., Charles C. Thomas, 1974, p. 93.

14. Picciano, M. F. and Guthrie, H. A.: Copper, iron, and zinc contents of mature human milk. *Am J Clin Nutr, 29*:242, 1976.

15. Altschule, M. D. and Smith, C. A.: Blood carbonic anhydrase activity in newborn infants and their mothers. *Pediat, 6*:717, 1950.

16. Smith, J. C., Jr., McDaniel, E. G., Fan, F. F., and Halsted, J. A.: Zinc: a trace element in vitamin A metabolism. *Science, 181*:954, 1973.

17. Abdulla, M.: Vitamin A deficiency, xerophthalmia and blindness. *Nutr Rev, 32*:350, 1974.

18. Henkin, R. I.: Zinc in wound healing. *N Engl J Med, 291*:675, 1974.

19. Low, W. I. and Ikram, H.: Plasma zinc in acute myocardial infarction. Diagnostic and prognostic implications. *Br Heart J, 38*:1339, 1976.

20. Halsted, J. A. and Smith, J. C., Jr.: Plasma zinc in health and disease. *Lancet, 1*:322, 1970.

21. Crawford, L. L. and Connor, J. D.: Zinc and hippocampal function. *J Orthomol Psychiatr, 4*:39, 1975.

22. Michaelsson, G., Juhlin, L., and Vahlquist, A.: Effects of oral zinc and vitamin A in acne. *Arch Dermatol, 113*:31, 1977.

23. Klevay, L. M.: Coronary heart disease: the zinc/copper hypothesis. *Am J Clin Nutr, 28*:764, 1975.
24. Margen, S. and King, J. C.: Effect of oral contraceptive agents on the metabolism of some trace minerals. *Am J Clin Nutr, 28*:392, 1975.
25. Prasad, A. S., Oberleas, D., Lei, K. Y., Moghissi, K. S., and Strayker, J. C.: Effect of oral contraceptive agents on nutrients: 1. Minerals. *Am J Clin Nutr, 28*:377, 1975.

CHROMIUM AND GLUCOSE
TOLERANCE FACTOR (GTF)

THE METAL CHROMIUM has recently come into prominence as an essential trace element in human nutrition. Although observations in animals began to point toward the role of chromium in intermediary metabolism about fifteen years ago, the evidence as regards man was not sufficiently impressive to encourage an extended discussion of chromium in the third edition of the Nutrition Foundation's *Present Knowledge in Nutrition*, published in 1967. The accumulation of information since that date is described in the excellent reviews by Hambridge[1] and Mertz.[2,3] The contents of these three articles comprise a thorough account of the extensive studies available in animals and their tissues. Accordingly, this need not be discussed here. The data obtained in man are far less abundant, but nevertheless permit some understanding of the way in which certain chromium compounds function.

Chromium is most abundant in whole grains and unrefined sugars, molasses containing by far the largest amounts. Milling grains and refining sugars remove almost all of the chromium. Although vegetables contain it, the practice of throwing away the cooking water causes large losses. Cows' milk contains very little of it, as does soy protein. It is evident that the diet of many American children and of some adults is very low in chromium. (Diets in the Middle East—excluding Egypt—and in some other parts of Africa are also low in chromium.) There is some evidence that eating carbohydrates from which the chromium has been removed increases the excretion of the metal from the body. In American adults the chromium content of the tissues is much lower than in younger persons. The decreases in tissue chromium content with age are striking. A question arises about whether this change is due to "aging" (whatever that is), or is owing to changing nutritional habits in the elderly.

The latter can clearly be implicated, but the former cannot be ruled out. The tissues of adult Americans contain far less chromium than that of starving African children, an alarming statistic, but one that cannot be evaluated. Pregnancy, especially closely spaced pregnancies, lowers the body chromium stores markedly.[4]

The role of chromium in human metabolism has been greatly clarified through the work of Mertz and his co-workers, as summarized by him in 1975.[3] The studies made to date indicate that the metal exists in two forms in the body. The first form comprises various coordinate compounds involving chlorine, water, and acetate as well as other organic acids, amino acids, sugars, and even vitamins. The published data include reports that these substances cause stimulation of activity of a number of enzyme systems, but these data must be accepted cautiously under present conditions of measurement which are designed specifically to exaggerate the function of enzyme systems. In none of these substances or activities does the chromium act as an essential dietary substance.

On the other hand, there is a type of chromium compound which clearly has specific biochemical effects as an essential nutritional substance. In this chromium compound—perhaps there is more than one—the chromium is trivalent, and it exists as a complex with nicotinic acid. This complex is given stability in the body by combining with certain amino acids. The chromium-nicotinic acid has been given the name *glucose tolerance factor* (GTF), a name that clearly expresses its known functions. It should probably be regarded as a vitamin, analogous perhaps to vitamin B_{12}, which consists of an organic portion bound to a metal (cobalt in the case of vitamin B_{12}) without which it cannot function. (Of course the functions of GTF and vitamin B_{12} are quite different.)

Chromium deficiency in animals seems to reproduce the effects of insulin deficiency: glycosuria, hyperglycemia, deficiency of hepatic glycogen deposition, and decreased incorporation of amino acids into protein. When exogenous insulin is injected, it produces less than the expected fall in blood sugar. The metabolic effects of chromium deficiency are greatly exaggerated in animals subjected to a variety of stresses. Giving chromium to deficient animals reverses the apparent diabetic condition; it also lowers the blood cholesterol level. Chromium supplementation of the diet protected ill-fed rats—the only species studied—against the deleterious effects of excessive physical activity and also decreased the mortality in animals that were bled to shock levels.[5]

Glucose tolerance factor evidently works in association with insulin. It seems to aid in the binding of insulin to cell membranes, both on and within the cells. For example, the binding of insulin to the mitochondrial membrane and the swelling of the mitochondria after insulin is administered are both potentiated by chromium. When glucose is given and insulin called forth, the serum chromium rises in normal subjects, but not in deficiency states.

As regards GTF, it is made slowly from administered inorganic chromium. GTF accumulates in the liver. There is a fairly good correlation between the concentrations of inorganic chromium and of GTF in foods, but inorganic chromium, whatever its source, cannot fully reproduce the action of GTF in conditions of chromium deficiency.

Chromium therapy has been tried in two types of disease in man. Inorganic chromium salts have been given to diabetics of all ages. It seems to be most effective in late, adult-onset diabetes, but not in all cases. It works very slowly and does not control the diabetes completely. Chromium has also been used in infantile protein-calorie deficiency. It improves the rate of removal of glucose from the circulation and, by increasing hepatic glycogen deposition, it prevents the hypoglycemia that characterizes the condition.

The evaluation of the state of chromium nutrition is difficult. The inorganic chromium content of foods is incompletely known, and moreover, it is not a satisfactory indication of the content of GTF, the active material. Measurement of the serum chromium level is technically difficult and may not be very informing. Measurements of hair chromium concentration are believed by some to be useful, but they have not been tried on a large scale.

RECOMMENDATIONS

Under present conditions it appears that an adequate diet (in the absence of stress) is the only guarantee against deficiency. This diet consists of yeast, beef, liver, whole grains, and crude unrefined sugar products. There is no need to eat molasses if the other foods are taken. If vegetables are to be an important source of chromium, they must be cooked without discarding the cooking water.

REFERENCES

1. Hambridge, K. M.: Chromium nutrition in man. *Am J Clin Nutr, 27*: 505, 1974.
2. Mertz, W.: Chromium occurrence and function in biological systems. *Physiol Rev, 49*:163, 1969.
3. Mertz, W.: Effects and metabolism of glucose tolerance factor. *Nutr Rev, 33*:129, 1975.
4. Mahalko, J. R. and Bennion, M.: The effect of parity and time between pregnancies on material hair chromium concentration. *Am J Clin Nutr, 29*:1069, 1976.
5. Mertz, W. and Roginski, E. E.: Effects of chromium (III) supplementation on growth and survival under stress in rats fed low protein diets. *J Nutr, 97*:531, 1969.

OTHER TRACE ELEMENTS

Recent reviews show that vanadium, nickel, and tin are essential for normal growth and function in mammals and birds.[1] There are no data in man, but there is no reason to doubt that they play a role in human physiology. Of these three, only vanadium need be considered as possibly being marginal or deficient in human diet. Of the common foods analyzed, eggs and rice contain by far the largest amounts, with other common foods combined yielding low values. Molybdenum is also an essential metal in some species, but there are no data for man.

Three nonmetals should also be considered: selenium, silicon, and fluoride. As regards selenium, there is a large amount of literature that describes its role as a biochemical antioxidant. In this capacity it seems to have at least a potential function as a partial replacement for vitamin E. This ambiguous role is made even more so by uncertainties about the function of vitamin E itself in man. Although the soils in some parts of this country contain large amounts of selenium—enough to poison grazing animals that eat the grasses there—there is nothing to indicate that selenium affects human nutrition.

Silicon is usually thought of as a thoroughly insoluble component of the rocks that make up most of the earth's dry surface. However, certain of its salts, the silicates, are freely soluble and are abundant in some vegetables. Eggs contain small amounts, but more than other animal foods. In mammals, silicon is an important constituent of some mucopolysaccharides that make up blood vessel walls.[1] The silicon content of the blood vessels and other tissues decreases with age. Atherosclerotic blood vessels are severely depleted of silicon, but whether this is cause or effect is not known.

The place of fluoride in human nutrition has recently been reviewed by Underwood.[2] Although the element has demonstrably favorable effects in the human body, there is no evidence that it is *essential*. There is no evidence that a deficiency of fluoride intake does any harm except to favor dental caries and osteoporosis. There is clearly a lower incidence not only of dental caries but of osteoporosis in persons who live in areas in which the water is rich in fluoride. Of the common foods, only fish contains appreciable amounts of fluoride. It must be borne in mind that the accumulated observations on fluoride in drinking water do not explain all situations in which very low incidences of dental caries occur in localized geographical areas. There are reports in which a low regional incidence is not associated with regional differences in fluoride content.[3] An excess of fluoride in water and food causes an extremely disabling disease, fluorosis, which is endemic in Asia.

REFERENCES

1. Nielsen, F. H. and Sandstead, H. H.: Are nickel, vanadium, silicon, and tin essential for man? A review. *Am J Clin Nutr,* 27:513, 1974.
2. Underwood, E. J.: *Trace Elements In Human And Animal Nutrition.* New York, Academic Press, 1971, p. 369.
3. Rothman, K. J., Glass, R. L., Esprinal, F., and Veley, H.: Caries-free teeth in the absence of the fluoride ion. *J Public Health Dent,* 32:225, 1972.

PART IV

VITAMINS

INTRODUCTION

THE EXISTENCE OF accessory food factors has been recognized for several centuries, and the identity of the individual vitamins known for decades. Nevertheless, specific biochemical roles of the vitamins, their metabolic fate in the body, and the mechanisms whereby they prevent (or reverse) the physiologic and anatomic manifestations of deficiencies are still incompletely known. Whereas our knowledge of thiamine and niacin is now both so extensive and so detailed as to have created much of today's biochemistry, information about the other vitamins is either specific for only one tissue (as in the case of vitamin A and the retina) or so fragmentary as to be confusing or useless. For example, how does it help the medical practitioner to know that vitamin B_6 deficiency impairs the synthesis of gamma-amino-butyric acid in the brain?; and so on.

Most of the known vitamins were discovered because they were found to play one or more highly specific and readily recognizable roles in clinical medicine (including pathology). However, most of them remain enigmas to the biochemist. This is most unfortunate because it has made it impossible for bio-chemists to develop clinical-laboratory methods of evaluating vitamin deficiencies—methods that might clarify many ambiguities of clinical practice.

Despite this lack of usable laboratory methods, physicians in those parts of the world where malnutrition is endemic have dealt with the problem of vitamin therapy fairly satisfactorily. Knowing which regional diets are deficient, and being able readily to diagnose the specific deficiencies by their overt typical clinical criteria, they are able to prescribe the necessary vitamin(s). Moreover, in these regions the deficiencies occur in patients whose total dietary intake is marginal (except perhaps for trace minerals) and in some cases the deficiency may be exacerbated and made overt by diarrheal or other febrile diseases endemic in these regions. Nevertheless, it is probable that physicians in these areas overlook many instances of mild vitamin deficiency.

In this country, on the other hand, except in children, whose nutritional needs are great, and except in some pockets of rural poverty off the beaten track, the majority of persons who might have vitamin deficiencies do not take a diet low in all components. In fact, hyperalimentation in terms of total calories and of calories derived from carbohydrate is likely to be prevalent. It may lead to a combination of obesity with specific malnutrition. In this setting, evaluation of vitamin status is more complicated and subtle than in some other areas. Accordingly, the physician who practices in our country must evaluate vitamin status by considering a number of factors that do not play important roles in developing countries.

The vitamin content—or at least the content of the known vitamins—of the average American diet is widely regarded as good —or even superb—in all respects. This conclusion is based only on published figures for recommended daily intakes of nutrients. These figures, which are meant to apply to "most healthy persons" clearly do not apply to some healthy persons or to persons who are under stress or who have illnesses, however minor. Moreover, after the superb American diet has been harvested, gathered, or slaughtered, it is prepared for sale in large volume and thereby loses much of its nutritional value. Recent studies indicate that 30 percent of the average American diet has no nutritional value other than calories.[1] In addition, clinical criteria, developed to diagnose severe deficiency states in persons whose total intake is marginal, may not apply in a population taking a normal diet or a grossly unbalanced diet. (In using the word *unbalanced* I am not making a moral judgment; I am merely referring to a diet materially different from the one that has kept our species in good health during the hundreds of thousands of years of its existence.)

Even if a diet seems to be adequate in vitamins, can we be sure that a person's vitamin status is healthy? The answer can only be an ambiguous "perhaps," for a number of reasons. (We shall omit discussing several self-evident causes of vitamin deficiencies despite adequate diets, e.g. congenitally increased requirements, pregnancy, malabsorption syndromes, liver disease, diabetes mellitus, effects of medication such as diphenylhydantoin in causing folate deficiency and of hydrazines in causing B_6 deficiency, etc. Nor need we discuss the loss of vitamins in cooking, especially in some frozen foods that have to be cooked a second time before being served.) Content does not insure availability. This is clearly established for some of the vitamins, as will be discussed later. However, this field has not been adequately studied. May antivitamin factors be present in the diet or are they made within the human body? We do not know whether this is important in man.

To what extent is an unbalanced diet important in the genesis of vitamin deficiencies? We know that giving thiamine alone to patients with B-complex deficiency may make overt a latent deficiency of one of the other of these vitamins. There is evidence also that a diet excessively high in purified carbohydrate may cause deficiencies of the B-complex vitamins. Another example is afforded by diets excessively high in polyunsaturated fats. Such diets are taken by three groups of normal persons: (1) infants fed on artificial formulas, (2) adults who find butter too expensive and who regularly use margarine instead, and (3) American adults who take large amounts of polyunsaturated fats for superstitious reasons. The excessive intake of polyunsaturated fats produces vitamin E deficiency. Since we have no clear account of the role of vitamin E in the human body economy, we do not know what symptoms to look for.

What about "enriched" foods? These are bread and cereal foods from which vitamins (and minerals) have been removed during preparation. The food elements known to have been removed are then replaced. These foods are adequate in vitamins —the labels say so. (Of course, the unidentified substances removed, if any, cannot be replaced.) However, at least some of the vitamins as they exist in the chemist's bottle are totally inert. They must be incorporated into enzymes or cofactors in the body before they can become active. Thus, some of the B-complex vitamins must be phosphorylated, e.g. thiamine becoming carboxylase and niacin becoming pyridine nucleotides. Whether there are hindrances to phosphorylation in some persons is not known. Moreover, the enzyme systems that incorporate the vitamins have cofactors that are as important as the vitamins. In the case of thiamine, one cofactor is lipoic acid. I have never seen a food label that stated that lipoic acid was present in or had been added to the food in adequate amounts.

These are some of the reasons that make a physician wonder whether apparently healthy people are adequately nourished with respect to vitamins. Since the water-soluble vitamins do not commonly have adverse side-effects, even in substantial amounts, physicians see no objection to their use by apparently normal persons in this country.

In addition, some attention should be paid to the factor of stress. But how is stress defined and measured in man? No unambiguous answer can be offered. Nevertheless, there is evidence that stress increases the need for at least some vitamins.

Thus far we have only talked about the use of vitamins to satisfy physiological or pathophysiological requirements. We must also consider the use of vitamins in pharmacological doses. The use of vitamins in these much larger doses is analogous to the use of adrenal corticoids in pharmacologic doses in patients in whom there is not the slightest indication of adrenal cortical insufficiency. The water-soluble vitamins rarely cause untoward reactions in large doses, and so the use of pharmacologic doses can be given without apprehension. One fat-soluble vitamin, vitamin D, has been used in pharmacologic doses to treat hypoparathyroidism, but the taking of large amounts of fat-soluble vitamins may be hazardous.

It is regrettable, but not surprising, that there is as yet no extensive coherent body of biochemical information that might help physicians to understand the vitamin deficiencies, except for rickets. It is also regrettable that most published clinical studies today involve populations either in maldeveloped countries where subsistence farming has been replaced by one-crop agriculture, or in economically depressed areas where total food intake is low, or in large cities where elderly and other unemployables congregate and subsist on meager stipends, the effective size of which may be diminished by the cost of alcohol to the drinker and his dependents. Physicians find the reported studies of little value in their practice. Consequently, despite the vast volume of the publications, the literature on vitamin nutrition in man can at best provide guidance but can never define the way to prevent or treat vitamin deficiencies.

Under the present circumstances, the practitioner is forced to rely on his own experience, that is, on trial and error, with the hope that the errors end not equal in number to the trials but substantially fewer.

As regards food as a source of vitamins—the so-called *natural* vitamins uncritically sought after by certain laymen—certain limitations must be borne in mind. The fat-soluble vitamins exist in food as such or as immediate precursors that usually, but not always, can be changed by the body to the vitamins. This change may not occur in disease. Vitamin C exists as such but is readily destroyed by oxidation as in cooking. Water-soluble vitamins, i.e. thiamine, niacin, pyridoxine, and folate cannot be absorbed as such from food. The first three exist in food as parts of enzyme systems, in combination with phosphate and sometimes other components. These vitamins must be stripped of these constituents before they can be absorbed from the intestinal tract. Once absorbed, however, they are inert until recombined into something resembling their original form. Either the separation or the reconstitution, or both, may not occur in some disease states. These vitamins may also be destroyed in cooking. Folate exists in nature conjugated with several glutamate moieties, and it must be separated from some of them before it can be absorbed. Vitamin B_{12} cannot be absorbed at all unless the gastrointestinal tract makes "intrinsic factor."

Moreover, it is known that several vitamins, i.e. A, D, and folate must be further changed chemically in the body before they can serve their metabolic function.

All these matters will be discussed in the sections on the individual vitamins. In the meantime, it is important to reiterate the general principles formerly stated: An internist who ignores nutritional factors in his patients cannot be considered competent except in a limited technical way; a nutritionist must be a well-trained internist.

REFERENCES

1. Hansen, R. G.: An index of food quality. *Nutr Rev, 31*:1, 1973.

VITAMIN A

Research on the physical chemistry of the visual pigments in the past few decades has been brilliantly successful. We now have a massive amount of information on the role of vitamin A in the action of these pigments and of the consequent detection and transmission of visual stimuli. This remarkable accumulation of data has permitted an understanding of the biochemistry of vision. It has also, regrettably, pushed far into the background important information that clinicians should have on the anatomical role of vitamin A in connective tissue formation (including the connective tissue of the eyeball in keratomalacia) and in maintaining the integrity of cuboidal, columnar, and pseudocolumnar epithelium in the urinary tract, the bronchi, and the lining and glands of the conjunctiva (where xerophthalmia manifests itself). The symptom of night blindness caused by lack of vitamin A in the visual pigment is far less serious a clinical manifestation than the other listed signs of vitamin A deficiency.

The effect of vitamin A deficiency on the epithelia listed is well known.[1] The deficiency produces squamous metaplasia, first patchy and then becoming extensive, in these epithelia. The areas of squamous metaplasia are highly susceptible to bacterial invasion, and stubborn infections often develop. So common were occurrences of this type that some early authors gave vitamin A a specific role as a preventive of all infections. Infections that develop in areas of vitamin A deficiencies will persist until the vitamin A deficiency that permitted their development is cured.

Evidence on the fact that vitamin A acts in collagen formation has appeared more recently. Extending earlier work of others, Ehrlich et al.[2] showed that vitamin A prevents the effects of glucocorticoids in retarding wound fibrosis. Moreover, vitamin A alone stimulates the growth and multiplication of fibroblasts and increases the formation of hydroxyproline, all resulting in

90

the accelerated laying down of collagen fibers. Vitamin A is also essential for spermatogenesis, and a deficiency of it may cause sterility.[3]

The manifestations of vitamin A deficiency include night blindness, i.e. impairment of dark adaptation. The often-described xerophthalmia is not common in this country, but examination with the slit-lamp will show the corneal cellular infiltration that marks its onset. Keratomalacia is rare in this country but appears to be not uncommon in developing countries. In our country, cutaneous perifollicular hyperkeratosis is easily recognized (although it is not specific for vitamin A deficiency). Patients with the deficiency develop thick stubborn calluses on the feet and sometimes in the elbows. Urine specimens obtained by catheterization contain squamous cells, an abnormal finding.

Much of what is considered vitamin A in the diet is not the vitamin at all. More than half—in some cases more than two thirds—of the so called vitamin A in the diet of Americans is really one carotene or another, chiefly the beta form. Carotene and vitamin A are widely distributed in the yellow vegetables and some leafy ones. Tomatoes are also a good source. Milk fats—including some cheeses—and fish liver oils are also excellent sources. As a rule, little of the vitamin and provitamin are lost in cooking, but prolonged or repeated cooking may induce significant losses. Vitamin A is usually ingested as an ester and is hydrolyzed in the gut. The absorption of the vitamin and provitamins requires bile acids.[1, 4] Hence, a bile-acid deficiency may impair absorption.[1, 4] This is true because a micellar phase must be present in the gut if absorption is to occur.[4] This implies that a very low total fat intake will also impair vitamin A absorption, and this is known to occur. Hence, vitamin A deficiency may occur despite a good intake of the vitamin if fat intake is markedly restricted. Protein intake must also be adequate, according to some studies.

According to present concepts, the vitamin A in food is retinol ester, and this yields retinol when hydrolyzed in the intestine. Retinol is absorbed and is transported in the lymph to the thoracic duct as retinol or as reconstituted retinol esters. Approximately 90 percent of the retinol is bound to a pre-albumin called retinol-binding protein (RBP). Retinol is stored in the liver and released under the influence of zinc (see page 72). In at least some tissues the active form of the vitamin is retinal, the aldehyde formed from retinol by alcohol dehydrogenase. This transformation cannot occur if alcohol is present.[4] Some of the intestinal carotene is changed to vitamin A in the intestinal wall. The rest is absorbed unchanged, but some of this is changed to vitamin A in the liver.

In starving persons, the serum levels of beta-carotene and retinol esters fall. Patients with anorexia nervosa show surprising deviations from this finding,[5] for the serum level of beta-carotene is greatly elevated, and the levels of all the measured vitamin A forms, retinyl esters, retinol, and retinoric acid are also high. There is no explanation for this peculiarity, but it may be used diagnostically.

The vitamin A status of patients with malabsorption has interested physicians for some time. Serum vitamin A levels after a test meal have been used in diagnosis. The vitamin A status varies with the cause of the malabsorption and, hence, is useless as a general diagnostic measure.[6] It has been so used in ascaris infestation, where malabsorption has been found.[7] In patients with intestinal disease who showed great increases in stool fat and also impairment of xylose absorption, the serum retinol and retinol-binding protein are normal. On the other hand, children with cystic fibrosis or with celiac disease often show decreased serum levels of vitamin A as do also patients with tropical or nontropical sprue. However, even in these conditions there is much overlap with the normal. A number of other clinical conditions have been found to affect vitamin A transport.[8] Thus, liver disease, both acute and chronic, and hyperthyroidism cause low serum vitamin A levels, due apparently to low levels of retinol-binding protein. In severe chronic renal disease, the concentration of this protein is very high, and the vitamin A level rises with it. Studies of vitamin A levels are of little value as diagnostic aids in malnutrition.

Estrogen causes a change in vitamin A status, as evidenced by the findings before and after starting certain oral contraceptives.[9, 10, 11] The serum vitamin A level rises and that of beta-carotene falls, a phenomenon that suggests increased transformation of the provitamin to the vitamin. The situation in pregnancy is complicated by increased needs for vitamin A and the free use of nutritional supplements.[12]

As already noted, most of our intake of what is called vitamin A is usually in the form of the provitamin, carotene. Is it possible that vitamin A deficiency can arise through inadequate transformation of carotene to vitamin A? This has been discussed in the past.[13] It is common in myxedema and may occur in diabetes mellitus. I believe that this disorder occurs more frequently in diabetic patients than is usually recognized. In diabetes mellitus, very high serum carotene levels occur frequently, and some of the patients show readily visible signs of vitamin A deficiency in the form of perifollicular hyperkeratosis over the trunk and proximal parts of the extremities and also very thick and resistant calluses on the feet and elbows. This is remarkable because the patients usually take a high carotene diet with relatively small amounts of vitamin A.

It is clear that serum levels of vitamin A (or of carotene) give no true indication of the hepatic and other stores. They similarly give no true indication of the utilization of the vitamin. In addition, vitamin A, however richly deposited in liver stores, is not available for body use in zinc deficiency (page 72). Moreover, dietary estimates may be misleading in sprue, perhaps in cystic fibrosis and in celiac disease. The same is true of patients taking cholestyramine, mineral oil (as a bowel lubricant or as a constituent of low calorie salad dressing), colchicine, or neomycin.[14]

Vitamin A toxicity is a danger when large doses are taken or when moderately large doses are taken over a period of months. In addition it may occur on a dietary basis from eating the livers of some wild animals.

RECOMMENDATIONS

Patients who have a deficient intake of vitamin A should, of course, receive a daily supplement of 5,000 units. This should be doubled in pregnant women.

Patients who have a deficient intake of the vitamin or who cannot transform carotene into the vitamin and who have stubborn infections of the urinary tract or of the bronchi should receive 25,000 units of pure vitamin A per day for a month, and then 5,000 to 10,000 units a day indefinitely. A water-soluble preparation is advisable.

Vitamin A, like the other fat-soluble vitamins, may be toxic in high doses, and care must be taken to detect toxicity if it occurs.

REFERENCES

1. Altschule, M. D.: Vitamin A deficiency in spite of adequate diet in congenital atrasia of the bile ducts and jaundice. *Arch Pathol, 20*:845, 1935.
2. Ehrlich, H. P., Tarver, H., and Hunt, T. K.: Effects of vitamin A and glucocorticoids upon inflammation and collagen synthesis. *Ann Surg, 177*:222, 1973.
3. Van Thiel, D. H., Gavaler, J., and Lester, R.: Ethanol inhibition of vitamin A metabolism in the tester: possible mechanism for sterility in alcoholics. *Science, 186*:941, 1974.
4. Barnard, D. L. and Heaton, K. W.: Bile acids and vitamin A absorption in man: the effects of two bile acid-binding agents, cholestyramine and liquin. *Gut, 14*:316, 1973.
5. Robboy, M. S., Sato, A. S., and Schwabe, A. D.: The hypercarotinemia in anorexia nervosa: a comparison of vitamin A and carotene levels in various forms of menstrual dysfunction and cachexia. *Am J Clin Nutr, 27*:362, 1974.
6. Smith, F. R. and Lundenbaum, J.: Human serum retinol transplant in malabsorption. *Am J Clin Nutr, 27*:700, 1974.
7. Mahalanabis, D., Julan, K. N., Maitra, T. K., and Agarwal, S. K.: Vitamin A absorption in ascariasis. *Am J Clin Nutr, 29*:1372, 1976.
8. Smith, F. R. and Goodman, DeW. S.: The effects of diseases of the liver, thyroid, and kidneys on the transport of vitamin A in human plasma. *J Clin Invest, 50*:2426, 1971.
9. Prasad, A. S., Lei, K. Y., Oberleas, D., Morghissi, K. S., and Stryker, J. C.: Effect of oral contraceptive agents on nutrients: II. Vitamins. *Am J Clin Nutr, 28*:385, 1975.
10. Young, D. L. and Chan, P. L.: Effects of a progestogen and a sequential type of oral contraceptive on plasma vitamin A, vitamin E, cholesterol and triglycerides. *Am J Clin Nutr, 28*:686, 1975.
11. Young, D. L.: Relationships between cigarette smoking, oral contraceptives, and plasma vitamins A, E, C, and plasma triglycerides and cholesterol. *Am J Clin Nutr, 29*:1216, 1976.

12. Gal, I. and Parkinson, C. E.: Effects of nutrition and other factors on pregnant women's serum vitamin A levels. *Am J Clin Nutr*, 27:688, 1974.
13. Cohen, H.: Observations on carotenemia. *Ann Intern Med*, 28:219, 1958.
14. Gaginalla, T. S.: Drug-induced malabsorption. *Drug Ther*, December 1975, p. 88.

THIAMINE – VITAMIN B₁

T HIAMINE DEFICIENCY probably has occurred sporadically since man's earliest days on earth. However, it became a widespread disease, with victims in the hundreds of thousands, when the rice-milling industry spread across Asia. It was probably the first example of how injudicious food processing, a consequence of the industrialization of the food industry, can bring disaster to populations of marginal economic status. The discovery that beriberi was due to dietary deficiency was an accomplishment of Japanese naval medicine. The later working out of the vitamin's roles in bodily functions stimulated the theory and practice of modern biochemistry to an enormous degree. Modern biochemistry is unimaginable without knowledge of where and how thiamine works.

The vitamin's structure is known. Thiamine consists of a pyrimidine ring joined to a thiazole ring by a methylene bridge. The bridge is a weak link and is easily broken by heating, especially at an alkaline pH. Grain and cereal foods may lose much of their thiamine in milling. Moreover, the vitamin is freely soluble in water and is readily washed out during cooking in water. Accordingly, what seems to be a diet adequate in thiamine may, by the time it reaches the table, be markedly deficient. In addition, after absorption, considerable amounts of thiamine may be lost in the sweat. Some meats, especially pork, may be rich in the vitamin. It is possible also that we may gain some thiamine owing to the activity of intestinal bacteria, some of which synthesize the vitamin. When thiamine is given by rectum to human subjects, it appears in the urine, proving that it had been absorbed. In the same vein are experiments that show that the apparent "thiamine-sparing" effect of feeding ascorbic acid to rats is due to the stimulation of thiamine synthesis by intestinal bacteria.[1] On the other hand, thiamine may be inactivated by being split at the methylene bridge by the thiaminase present

96

in some foods, particularly raw fish and shellfish. However, an excess of thiamine appears to inactivate the enzyme, and it is probable that thiaminase is of little importance in the American diet. The requirement for thiamine is linked to the intake of carbohydrate.

The biochemical roles of thiamine have been extensively studied. Thiamine, when phosphorylated, becomes the enzyme cocarboxylase, required for the decarboxylation of the keto acids, pyruvate, and alpha-ketoglutarate. The reaction with pyruvate leads to the formation of acetyl-CoA, which then enters the Krebs cycle. (The decarboxylation of pyruvate also requires the nicotinic-acid containing nicotinamide-adenine-diphosphate, the pantothenic-acid containing coenzyme A, and thioctic acid.) The same enzyme is also a cofactor in the transketolase reaction.

The absorptions of thiamine hydrochloride, the form in which it exists commercially, and thiamine pyrophosphate, the form found in food, are limited. However, divided intake through the day increases the total that can be absorbed. Because of the limited absorbability of thiamine hydrochloride, attempts have been made to develop thiamine derivatives that more readily pass the mucosal barrier in the intestine.[2] Two lipid soluble compounds have been studied; these are thiamine propyl disulfide and thiamine tetrahydrofurfuryl disulfide. They are both absorbed much more completely than the hydrochloride and pyrophosphate and enter the red blood cells and spinal fluid much more readily.[2] The thiamine propyl disulfide has an unpleasant smell and, hence, cannot be used, but thiamine tetrahydrofurfuryl disulfide may prove to be an excellent compound to use when large amounts are required by mouth.

Evaluation of the thiamine status in man is not an accurate procedure. Although the blood pyruvate level rises in thiamine deficiency, an identical change occurs in many other conditions (see page 27). The blood levels of thiamine and thiamine pyrophosphate are also not useful because they may show only small decreases in conditions of serious thiamine deficiency. The same is true of the urine output of thiamine, measured usually as its derivative, thiochrome. This measurement is indicative of current thiamine intake and not of tissue thiamine level and so is not usable as a test of thiamine nutrition. A test that has come into favor recently is the measurement of the erythrocyte transketolase activity. The activity of this enzyme requires thiamine pyrophosphate. In some cases the erythrocyte transketolase activity may be measured before and after the addition of thiamine pyrophosphate, a significant increase being taken as evidence of the existence of a deficiency of thiamine. In addition, in some studies, bioassays using the growth of a microorganism have been used. Using the thiamine pyrophosphate stimulation test studies in patients with beriberi gives definitely abnormal values.[3] However, 10 or 15 percent of both healthy and sick children also give abnormal tests. In a study made in America, the values were found to vary with the red blood cell count, but the level in Negroes was lower than in whites.[4] It is known that the requirement for thiamine increases particularly during the third trimester of pregnancy. This is probably due to sequestration of the vitamin in the fetus, for umbilical cord blood contains a higher concentration than the mother's blood.[5] Both the blood and spinal fluid thiamine levels are low in alcoholic patients. Of course the erythrocyte transketolase values are also low in these patients. All rise with surprisingly little refeeding.[6]

In this country, thiamine deficiency occurs commonly in alcoholics and also in patients fed intravenously with glucose solutions for more than a week or ten days. A deficiency may also occur in patients with congestive heart failure who eat poorly and receive certain diuretics frequently. It may also be found in diabetics who perhaps do not phosphorylate thiamine normally after absorption. It also occurs in young women and girls who foolishly feed on sweets. Except for paresthesias, there are usually no signs of neuropathy in any but the alcoholics, who may, in extreme cases, develop Wernicke-Korsakoff's syndrome or else beriberi heart disease. The latter is easily recognized by the signs of vasodilatation, uncommon in most other types of congestive heart failure, and by the response to thiamine injections. In ordinary practice most patients encountered with thiamine deficiency experience extreme fatigability, owing to their Krebs cycle disorder, and a nervous depression the exact mechanism of which is not evident. In any case, the symptoms rapidly disappear when thiamine is given by injection in a dose of 10 mg.

Since giving one B vitamin may precipitate a deficiency of the other B vitamins, it is well to give a B-complex preparation.

Thiamine pyrophosphate is a cofactor in the activity of the enzyme alpha-keto-glutarate:glyoxylate carboligase, and hence it might be expected that urinary excretion of oxalate might be increased in a deficiency state. However, this does not occur for some unknown reason.[7]

There are few data on possible changes in thiamine metabolism in stress. There is one remarkable report of the decrease, in fact almost the total disappearance, of thiamine from the urine of deep-sea divers, the other vitamin measurements remaining unchanged.[8]

Thiamine deficiency is included in the problems created by drinking alcohol. In large part this is due to deficient intake of the vitamin. Perhaps the fact that alcohol in some way is metabolized as carbohydrate increases the need for the vitamin. Moreover, alcoholics with liver disease are unable to obtain much of the vitamin from natural food sources, such as yeast.[9] This is perhaps owing to an ability to dephosphorylate the natural vitamin in order to prepare it for absorption. However, alcoholics also absorb synthetic thiamine hydrochloride poorly.[10] What thiamine does get into the liver is likely to be drained out when the blood passing through the liver contains large amounts of alcohol, according to one report[11] but not another.[12]

RECOMMENDATIONS

There are no recorded toxic manifestations of thiamine. Sensitivity is reported as a rare occurrence after repeated, temporally spaced intravenous injections. The therapeutic dose is 50 to 200 mg by subcutaneous injection daily for a few days in overt thiamine deficiency.

Patients with subclinical B-vitamin deficiency, e.g. those with chronic congestive heart failure treated with some of the known diuretics, may well have deficiency changes in the terminal ileum. At any rate, they do not respond to oral vitamins and should receive an intramuscular injection of a B-vitamin mixture that contains 10 mg of thiamine twice a month indefinitely. Some diabetics seem to utilize the B vitamins poorly and do well when receiving an oral B-complex preparation daily. It is unfortunately a fact that in almost all cases diabetic neuropathy is due to vascular disease of the vasa nervora, and this syndrome does not respond to thiamine. However, the vitamin should be tried in such cases as it can do no harm.

Patients who live on intravenous feedings of glucose should receive the vitamin daily in doses of at least 10 mg.

Alcoholic patients constitute a special group. Their high thiamine requirement owing to high carbohydrate intake, their low dietary thiamine and poor absorption of the vitamin, and their losses while drinking suggest that their daily intake should be ten or twenty times the recommended daily intake. (This applies to riboflavin and niacin as well.)

REFERENCES

1. Murdock, D. S., Donaldson, M. I., and Gabler, C. J.: Studies on the mechanism of the "thiamine-sparing" effect of ascorbic acid in rats. *Am J Clin Nutr*, 27:696, 1974.
2. Baker, H., Thomson, A. D., Frank, O., and Leevy, C. M.: Absorption and passage of fat- and water-soluble thiamine derivatives into erythrocytes and cerebrospinal fluid of man. *Am J Clin Nutr*, 27:676, 1974.
3. Pongpanich, B., Strikrikkrich, N., Dhanametta, S., and Valyasevi, A.: Biochemical detection of thiamine deficiency in infants and children in Thailand. *Am J Clin Nutr*, 27:1399, 1974.
4. Warnock, L. G., Nichoaldi, G. E., and Burkhalter, V. J.: Erythrocyte transketolase levels in a high school population by sex and ethnic group. *Am J Clin Nutr*, 27:905, 1974.
5. Bamji, M. S.: Enzymic evaluation of thiamine, riboflavin, and pyridoxine status of parturient women and their newborn infants. *Br J Nutr*, 35:259, 1976.
6. Dastur, D. K., Santhadevi, N., Quadros, E. V., Avari, F. C. R., Wadia, N. H., Desai, M. M., and Bharucha, E. P.: The B-vitamins in malnutrition with alcoholism. *Br J Nutr*, 26:143, 1976.
7. Salyer, W. R. and Salyer, D. C.: Thiamine deficiency and oxalosis. *Am J Clin Pathol*, 27:558, 1974.
8. Frattali, V. and Robertson, R.: Nutritional evaluation of humans during an oxyglu-helium dive to a simulated depth of 1,000 feet. *Aerosp Med*, 44:14, 1973.
9. Baker, H., Frank, O., Zetterman, R. K., Rajan, K. S., ten Hove, W., and Leevy, C. M.: Inability of chronic alcoholics to use food as a

source of folates, thiamine and vitamin B_6. *Am J Clin Nutr, 28*: 1377, 1975.

10. Thomson, A. D., Baker, H., and Leevy, C. M.: Patterns of [33]S-thiamine hydrochloride absorption in the malnourished alcoholic patient. *J Lab Clin Med, 76*:34, 1970.

11. Sorrell, M. F., Baker, H., Barak, A. J., and Frank, O.: Release by ethanol of vitamins into rat liver perfusates. *Am J Clin Nutr, 27*:743, 1974.

12. Frank, O., Linsada-Opper, A., Sorrell, M. F., Zetterman, R., and Baker, H.: Effects of a single intoxicating dose of ethanol on the vitamin profile of organelles in rat liver and brain. *J Nutr, 106*:606, 1976.

RIBOFLAVIN

T HE SCIENTIFIC LITERATURE contains reports of a large amount of work on the nutritional aspects of dietary riboflavin in animals and on the enzymiology of the vitamin in isolated tissues. These unfortunately are so variable, contradictory, and incomplete[1] as to preclude using this material to elucidate clinical phenomena in man. The conditions of utilization of riboflavin in man are not completely known. It is known, however, that there is an increased requirement for the vitamin later in pregnancy, probably owing to its sequestration in the fetus.[2]

The changes described as typical of riboflavin deficiency consist in greasy scaling of the skin at the mucosal-cutaneous borders, especially the corners of the mouth. The skin of the paranasal creases and the adjacent cheeks is also said to be commonly involved. However, patients found to have low serum or urine concentrations of the vitamin often show no skin changes whatever.[3, 4] Even when riboflavin deficiency is produced experimentally in human subjects, there may be no external evidences of it.[5] Riboflavin deficiency has also been shown to cause behavioral abnormalities. There is nothing specific about these clinical measurements. They may precede the more specific clinical signs of riboflavin deficiency.[6] This unsatisfactory state of affairs, together with the finding that serum and urine levels change quickly in response to short-term changes in nutrition, has led to a search for more reliable laboratory methods. One has apparently been found. It is based on the fact that the red blood cell enzyme, glutathione reductase, requires the riboflavin derivative, flavin adenine dinucleotide. The test gives abnormal results in many alcoholic patients, despite the absence of all clinical evidences of the deficiency.[3, 7] In passing, it should be noted that alcoholic patients absorb riboflavin readily (unlike some other vitamins), and so their commonly found riboflavin deficiency must be due to poor dietary habits.[8]

In riboflavin deficiency, one cannot expect definitive help from routine laboratory studies. One must rely on the history of dietary inadequacy due to ignorance, to alcoholism, or to liver or gastrointestinal disease.

RECOMMENDATIONS

If there is any question of deficiency of any B vitamin except folate or B_{12}, the patient should take 10 mg of riboflavin daily. There are no toxic effects with even very large doses.

REFERENCES

1. Mickelsen, O.: Present knowledge of riboflavin. In *Present Knowledge in Nutrition*. New York, The Nutrition Foundation, Inc. 1967, p. 61.
2. Bamji, M. S.: Enzymic evaluation of thiamine, riboflavin and pyridoxine status of parturient women and their newborn infants. *Br J Nutr*, 35:259, 1976.
3. Leevy, V. M., Baker, H., Ten Hove, W., Frank, O., and Cherrick, G. R.: B-Complex vitamins in liver disease of the alcoholic. *Am J Clin Nutr*, 16:335, 1965.
4. Rosenthal, W. S., Adham, N. F., Lopez, R., and Cooperman, J. M.: Riboflavin deficiency in complicated chronic alcoholism. *Am J Clin Nutr*, 26:858, 1973.
5. Tillotson, J. A. and Baker, E. M.: An enzymatic measurement of the riboflavin status in man. *Am J Clin Nutr*, 25:425, 1972.
6. Sterner, R. T. and Price, W. R.: Restricted riboflavin: within subject behavioral effects in humans. *Am J Clin Nutr*, 26:150, 1973.
7. Dastur, D. K., Santhadevi, N., Quadros, E. V., Avari, F. C. R., Wadia, N. H., Desai, M. M., and Bharucha, E. P.: The B-vitamins in malnutrition with alcoholism. *Br J Nutr*, 36:143, 1976.
8. Baker, H., Frank, O., Zetterman, R. K., Rajan, K. S., Ten Hove, W., and Leevy, C. M.: Inability of chronic alcoholics with liver disease to use food as a source of folates, thiamine, and vitamin B_6. *Am J Clin Nutr*, 28:1377, 1975.

NICOTINIC ACID (NIACIN)

Nicotinic acid, or niacin as it is usually called, was first discovered a century ago as a derivative of nicotine. Fifty years later it began to be thought of as a vitamin, and in 1938 it was identified as the pellagra-preventive factor. This came at a good time, for pellagra had become endemic not only in Europe but in America from Illinois south.

Endemic pellagra was a man-made disease, and the history of its occurrence as one-crop farming replaced subsistence farming is a sad example of man's inhumanity to man, as the articles by Roe[1] and Darby et al.[2] show. Endemic pellagra was a disease of people who fed on little other than cornmeal. (In this country they also ate pork fat and molasses.) Corn is a poor source of niacin and also of its precursor, tryptophan. The Central American Indian cultures that depended on corn were free of pellagra for two reasons: (1) they ate considerable amounts of beans and other vegetables and (2) they treated their corn with lime, thereby freeing what niacin there was from combination and making it available for utilization.

Niacin participates in almost all mammalian enzymic reactions as a cofactor. In the form of its amide, nicotinamide, it exists combined with adenine di- or triphosphate. (These compounds were formerly called diphospho- and triphosphopyridine nucleotides.)

Niacin differs from other vitamins in that man can synthesize it. Its source is tryptophan, and it is said that 60 milligrams of the amino acid ordinarily will yield one of niacin. However, this figure is not universally accepted, and it clearly does not apply in all conditions.[3] At any rate, the biochemistry of niacin is tied to that of tryptophan. Ingested tryptophan goes down several metabolic pathways. In the intestine, the amino acid may have its side chain removed by bacterial action, the indole residue becoming chiefly skatole. Some of the unchanged tryptophan absorbed from the gut is incorporated into tissue protein.

Some of the absorbed tryptophan is hydroxylated and deaminated to become serotonin and, thereafter, other amines.

Another portion is acted upon by tryptophan pyrollase, destroying the indole nucleus and forming kynurenine. Thence it may follow one of two paths. One ends as kynurenic and xanthurenic acids. The other pathway goes through anthranilic acid to nicotinic acid. The nicotinic acid then becomes a nucleotide and undergoes additional metabolic changes to methylnicotinamide, quinolic acid, etc.[2] It is apparent that only a small part of the ingested tryptophan goes to nicotinic acid. The kynurenine pathway requires vitamin B_6, and hence, a deficiency of that vitamin may, in rare cases, cause pellagra.[4] The vitamin is not stored in any great amount, and losses easily occur.

The clinical features of pellagra as encountered in the sporadic form in ordinary circumstances in America do not usually take the form of the extreme disease—diarrhea, dermatitis, dementia. In its early stages it may not be recognized at all by the unprepared physician. As Grace Goldsmith made clear in her perceptive clinical writings, the earliest evidence of pellagra is an agitated depression. If the patient avoids going out-of-doors, as is the habit of depressed persons, the dermatitis may never develop. Only the somewhat edematous beefy tongue suggests the diagnosis. A little later, confusion develops and, if elderly, the patient may be put away for life as senile.

The requirement for niacin is linked to caloric intake. In healthy persons it is said to be around 7 milligrams per day per thousand calories eaten.[2] However, some niacin in food is bound and unavailable for utilization.[5] The requirement is increased by the ingestion of leucine, a main constituent of the millet eaten by peasants in India.[6] Apparently leucine interferes with the action of pyridoxine[7] in the latter's role in the generation of niacin from tryptophan.

There seems to be no good way to measure niacin deficiency in man. Although the serum tryptophan level is low in pellagra, this is not a constant finding, and the differences are not great.[6] The urinary excretion of niacinamide metabolites may yield confusing results.[8] There are methods of measuring the niacin content of the blood, but they are cumbersome and not readily available. The diagnosis must be made clinically. Although endemic pellagra no longer exists in this country, owing largely to social rather than public health factors, sporadic pellagra still occurs. I have seen it in diabetics, in alcoholics, in elderly or mentally disturbed persons living alone, and in postoperative patients receiving the empty calories of intravenous glucose. In the last two conditions, there is evidently an imbalance between caloric and niacin intakes. As regards diabetes, there is evidence of impairment of the tryptophan-niacin pathway.[9] Recent work on experimental diabetes in animals confirms this.[10] In addition, it must be borne in mind that interference with the action of niacin may be owing to other changes in intermediary metabolism in diabetes. As regards alcoholics, not only are they likely to take a diet, including the alcohol, overloaded with empty calories, but they lose some of their liver stores of niacin when they drink.[11, 12] At any rate, the concentration of niacin in the blood and the cerebrospinal fluid may be very low in malnourished alcoholics.[13]

The status of niacin nucleotides is always changed by stress and by alcohol, both of which put the nucleotides in an oxidized state. This is harmful because a multitude of biochemical processes depend on the free change between oxidized and reduced states, and maintaining the oxidized states may change metabolic processes greatly. At the moment there is nothing to indicate that giving niacin can abolish this abnormal state.

The possibility that severe niacin depletion may interfere with the action of chromium, and thereby impair carbohydrate metabolism, is purely theoretical. Nevertheless, because the active form of chromium is a nicotinate (see page 77), the possibility cannot be dismissed. Future work should clarify this matter.

RECOMMENDATIONS

For the confused pellagrin: intramuscular B complex, three injections spread over five or six days. Each injection should contain of nicotinamide—20 mg, and of thiamine and riboflavin—10 mg each. Thereafter, oral medication of similar potency should be given daily. Chronic alcoholic patients should have 1 to 2 grams a day of niacinamide (plus other vitamins).

Niacin in doses of 100 mg or more may have uncomfortable side effects. (Despite this, it has been given in doses of 3.0 grams a day to lower the blood cholesterol level in futile attempts to slow the progression of atherosclerosis.) Niacinamide is tolerable in larger doses, although above 4.0 grams a day may cause rashes and mildly abnormal liver function tests.

The vitamin is not stored in any great amount, and losses easily occur.

REFERENCES

1. Roe, D. A.: The sharecropper's plague. *Natural History, 83*:52, 1974.
2. Darby, W. J., McNutt, K. W., and Todhunter, E. N.: Niacin. *Nutr Rev, 33*:289, 1975.
3. Vivian, V. M.: Relation between tryptophan-niacin metabolism and changes in nitrogen balance. *J Nutr, 82*:395, 1964.
4. Roe, D. A.: Drug-induced deficiency of B vitamins. *NY State J Med, 71*:2270, 1971.
5. Mason, J. B., Gibson, N., and Kodicek, E.: The chemical nature of the bound nicotinic acid of wheat bran. *Br J Nutr, 30*:297, 1973.
6. Ghafoorunissa and Rao, B. S. N.: Plasma amino acid pattern in pellagra. *Am J Clin Nutr, 28*:325, 1975.
7. Krishnaswamy, K., Rao, S. B., Raghuram, T. C., and Srikantia, S. G.: Effects of vitamin B$_6$ on leucine-induced changes in human subjects. *Am J Clin Nutr, 29*:177, 1976.
8. Consolazio, C. F., Johnson, H. L., Kozywicki, H. J., and Witt, N. I.: Tryptophan-niacin interrelationships during acute fasting and caloric restriction in man. *Am J Clin Nutr, 25*:572, 1972.
9. Rosen, D. A., Mengwyn, D., Becker, B., Stone, H. H., and Friedenwald, J. S.: Xanthurenic acid studies in diabetics with and without retinopathy. *Proc Soc Exp Biol Med, 88*:520, 1955.
10. Akarte, N. R. and Shastir, N. Y.: Studies on tryptophan-niacin metabolism in streptozotocin diabetic rats. *Diabetes, 25*:977, 1974.
11. Sorrell, M. F., Baker, N., Barak, A. J., and Frank, O.: Release by ethanol of vitamins into rat liver perfusates. *Am J Clin Nutr, 27*:743, 1974.
12. Frank, O., Linsada-Opper, A., Sorrell, M. F., Zetterman, R., and Baker, H.: Effects of a single intoxicating dose of ethanol on the vitamin profile of organelles in rat liver and brain. *J Nutr, 106*:606, 1976.
13. Dastur, D. K., Santhadevi, N., Quadros, E. V., Avari, F. C. R., Wadia, N. H., Desai, M. M., and Bharucha, E. P.: The B-vitamins in malnutrition with alcoholism. *Br J Nutr, 36*:143, 1976.

FOLIC ACID

Folates are widely distributed in food. However, they may be destroyed by cooking. Folates in food usually occur as poly-glutamates, i.e. pteroylglutamic acid with more than one glutamic acid side chain. After oral administration these food folates are deconjugated in the gut, yielding mono- or diglutamates. However, it must be borne in mind that keeping meat at close to room temperature or keeping ground meat at 5 degrees C for forty-eight hours will permit the enzyme in the meat to change the poly- to monoglutamates.[1] The enzymic deconjugation of food folates is the precursor of folate absorption into the blood.[2] The pH of the intestinal contents affects folate absorption, higher pH values depressing it.[3]

There may be several different causes of nutritional folate deficiency, viz., inadequate intake, inadequate deconjugation of food folate, and impaired absorption due to intestinal disease. In addition, folate deficiency may occur owing to increased tissue needs (as in pregnancy) or distorted metabolism of the vitamin.

Synthetic folic acid is readily absorbed from the intestine.[4] In fact, in some circumstances it may be absorbed better than the natural folic acid found in food. Folate is present in large amounts in vegetables, and hence, vegetarians usually have normal or even high serum values.[5] Seemingly low plasma values may be found in apparently healthy persons, more commonly women than men, and more commonly poor than well off.[6] The significance of plasma levels is not settled, first, because low values can occur without symptoms, and second, because plasma and bone-marrow concentrations correlate poorly with each other.[7] Moreover, serum and red blood cell folate concentrations do not always go together in patients who have anemias due to combined deficiencies. In iron deficiency, serum folate level is often low and red blood cell folate concentration is elevated.[8] Conversely, in vitamin B_{12} deficiency, red blood cell folate levels are low, and

108

serum folate concentrations are elevated.[9] Evidently vitamin B_{12} is necessary for the transfer of folate from the blood plasma to the cells. The serum folate level may change rapidly in response to feeding or depletion, but the red blood cell folate level is a better guide to saturation. Instead of relying on serum levels, which may be misleading, some physicians use a method that measures the absorption of ingested radioactively tagged folate.[10] This test is analogous to the Schilling test for the absorption of vitamin B_{12}. However, it measures absorption only and does not reveal the actual state of folic acid nutrition.

Patients who have had a subtotal gastrectomy may develop a type of small-intestinal malabsorption (perhaps associated with the dumping syndrome). Approximately one patient in three has a low serum folate level, but when this is not accompanied by iron or vitamin B_{12} deficiency (it usually is), the patients are usually not anemic.[11] Although failure to take a good diet is often a factor in postgastrectomy folate deficiency,[12] impaired absorption is an important factor in about 25 percent of the cases.[10] Impaired absorption is also found in celiac disease,[2] steatorrhea,[10] and upper intestinal resections.[10]

The effect of systemic infection was recently discussed by Cook et al.,[13] who used a double-lumen jejunal tube in their studies. The form of the vitamin used was the synthetic variety— not a polyglutamate. Patients with lobar pneumonia or active pulmonary tuberculosis exhibited a marked decrease in the absorption of the vitamin from the intestine. This impairment of absorption might occur in all febrile states. It is regrettable that there are as yet no data on other types of stress.

Pregnancy is an important factor in the genesis of folate deficiency. Although poverty is a factor, milder degrees of deficiency, with little or no anemia, need not be related to low economic status.[14] Fortification of food with synthetic folic acid is highly effective in preventing or curing the folate deficiency of pregnancy.[15] The cause of this folate deficiency appears to be estrogen. This substance in oral contraceptive pills may also cause folate deficiency.[16, 17, 18] The deficiency is believed by some to be due to inhibition of polyglutamate deconjugase, thereby preventing the absorption of food folate.[16, 17] The author has seen megaloblastic anemia responsive to synthetic folate in postmenopausal women who had been taking estrogen over a period of years.

The widespread occurrence of folate deficiency in alcoholics is well known. However, in one series of markedly malnourished alcoholics studied in India, only a portion of the patients showed low serum values,[19] but this low figure might have been owing to simultaneous B_{12} deficiency, which may elevate the serum folate level. Part of this may be due to poor food habits and, perhaps, damage to the liver and the intestinal mucosa. However, it is known that alcoholics cannot absorb food polyglutamate folate but can absorb synthetic monoglutamate folate.[20] Also, the presence of alcohol in the blood perfusing the liver causes the loss of stored folate from that organ.[21] The vitamin cannot reenter liver stores as long as alcohol is in the blood. The clinical consequences of this fact are self-evident. The fact that these patients have normal serum levels of the enzyme folate conjugase tells us nothing about the enzyme in the intestinal lining.

A different type of impaired folate metabolism occurs in patients who take anticonvulsant drugs. Patients who receive these drugs develop low serum and cerebrospinal fluid folate levels.[22] Giving them synthetic folic acid (the monoglutamate) raises the serum folate level, but the folate does not enter the cerebrospinal fluid. Evidently ordinary folate cannot cross the blood-brain barrier. The data suggest that the anticonvulsive drugs depressed the intestinal folate deconjugase in a manner similar to the action of estrogen, as described above. In some experiments giving the reduced form of folate, 5-methyltetrahydrofolate, was followed by a rise in cerebrospinal fluid folate level. The folate therapy did not affect the clinical course of the epilepsy.

The basic pathophysiology of folate deficiency is believed to be a deficiency in DNA synthesis. This suggested to a group at the Massachusetts Institute of Technology that it would be appropriate to study lymphocytic function in patients with the vitamin deficiency. The results showed a depression of cell-mediated immunity, reversible by folate thereby, in these patients.

RECOMMENDATIONS

Patients with inadequate folate intake alone can respond to any form of folate. Patients in whom the deficiency is due to estrogen or to alcohol need synthetic folate (the monoglutamate form). If anemic, they should be given 3 or 4 mg daily for a month, and then 1 mg a day for some weeks, to be followed by 1 mg two or three times a week thereafter. If symptoms or signs of neuropathy develop during this treatment period, the diagnosis was wrong and the condition is really B_{12} deficiency. Patients given anticonvulsants may need the reduced form of folate, 5-methyltetrahydrofolate.

REFERENCES

1. Reed, B., Weir, D., and Scott, J.: The fate of folate polyglutamates in meat during storage and processing. *Am J Clin Nutr, 29*:1393, 1976.
2. Jägerstad, M., Dencker, H., and Westesson, A.-K.: The hydrolysis and fate of conjugated folates in man. *Scand J Gastroenterol, 11*:283, 1976.
3. MacKenzie, J. F. and Russell, R. I.: The effect of pH on folic acid absorption in man. *Clin Sci Mol Med, 51*:363, 1976.
4. Nelson, E. W., Streiff, R. R., and Cerda, J. J.: Comparative bio-availability of folate and vitamin C from a synthetic and a natural source. *Am J Clin Nutr, 28*:1014, 1975.
5. Armstrong, B. K., Davis, R. E., Nicol, D. J., van Merwyk, A. J., and Larwood, C. J.: Hematological, vitamin B_{12}, and folate studies in Seventh Day Adventist vegetarians. *Am J Clin Nutr, 27*:712, 1974.
6. Hall, C. A., Bardwell, S. A., Allen, E. S., and Rappazzo, M. E.: Variations in plasma folate levels among groups of healthy persons. *Am J Clin Nutr, 28*:854, 1975.
7. Trubowitz, S., Frank, O., and Baker, H.: Survey of vitamin B_{12} and folate in the serum and marrow of hospitalized patients. *Am J Clin Nutr, 27*:580, 1974.
8. Omer, A. N., Finlayson, D. C., Shearman, D. J. C., Samson, R. R., and Girdwood, R. H.: Plasma and erythrocyte folate in iron deficiency and folate deficiency. *Blood, 35*:821, 1970.
9. Cooper, B. A. and Lowenstein, L.: Relative folate deficiency of erythrocytes in pernicious anemia and its connection with cyanocobalamine. *Blood, 24*:502, 1964.
10. Elsborg, L. and Bostrup-Madsen, P.: Folic and absorption in various gastrointestinal disorders. *Scand J Gastroenterol, 11*:333, 1976.

11. Mahmud, K., Ripley, D., Swaim, W. R., and Doscherholmen, A.: Hematologic complications of partial gastrectomy. *Ann Surg, 177:* 432, 1973.
12. Bradley, E. L. and Isaacs, J.: Postresectional anemia. *Arch Surg, 111:* 844, 1976.
13. Cook, G. C., Morgan, J. O., and Hoffbrand, A. V.: Impairment of folate absorption by systemic bacterial infections. *Lancet,* 2:1416, 1974.
14. Lowenstein, L., Brunton, L., and Hsich, T.-S.: Nutritional anemia and megaloblastosis in pregnancy. *Can Med Assoc J,* 94:636, 1966.
15. Colman, N., Barker, M., Green, R., and Merz, J.: Prevention of folate deficiency in pregnancy by food fortification. *Am J Clin Nutr,* 27:339, 1974.
16. Streiff, R. A.: Folate deficiency and oral contraceptives. *JAMA, 214:* 105, 1970.
17. Necheles, T. F. and Snyder, L. M.: Malabsorption of folate polyglutamates associated with oral contraceptive therapy. *N Engl J Med, 282:*858, 1970.
18. Prasad, A. S., Lei, K. Y., Oberleas, D., Moghissi, K. S., and Stryker, J. C.: Effect of oral contraceptive agents on nutrients: II. Vitamins. *Am J Clin Nutr, 28:*385, 1975.
19. Dastur, D. K., Santhadevi, N., Quadros, E. V., Avari, F. C. R., Wadia, N. H., Desai, M. M., and Bharucha, E. P.: The B-vitamins in malnutrition with alcoholism. *Br J Nutr,* 36:143, 1976.
20. Mattson, R. H., Gallagher, B. B., Reynolds, E. H., and Glass, D.: Folate therapy in epilepsy. *Arch Neurol,* 29:78, 1973.
21. Sorrell, M. F., Baker, H., Barak, A. J., and Frank, O.: Release by ethanol of vitamins into rat liver perfusates. *Am J Clin Nutr,* 27: 743, 1974.
22. Gross, R. L., Reid, J. V. O., Newberne, P. M., Burgess, B., Marston, R., and Hift, W.: Depressed cell-mediated immunity in megaloblastic anemia due to folic acid deficiency. *Am J Clin Nutr, 28:*225, 1975.
23. Gross, R. L., Reid, J. V. O., Newberne, P. M., Burgess, B., Marston, R., and Hift, W.: Depressed cell-mediated immunity in megaloblastic anemia due to folate deficiency. *Am J Clin Nutr, 28:*225, 1975.

PYRIDOXINE – VITAMIN B₆

T HE ROLE OF pyridoxine, in the form of pyridoxal phosphate or pyridoxamine phosphate, in a vast array of enzymic reactions, continues to expand as research goes on. Starting with Williams's review in 1967,[1] one can follow in *Annual Review of Biochemistry* the bewildering accumulation of biochemical knowledge about this vitamin. However, the significance of this fascinating material for clinical practice is not great and can be covered under only a few headings. Despite the many different functions of pyridoxal enzymes in amino acid, carbohydrate, and fat synthesis and metabolism, the recognizable deficiency states refer to only a few malfunctions, and some cannot be reliably referred to any of them.

Pyridoxine is essential for the synthesis of gamma-aminobutyric acid, a principal inhibitory brain substance. A lack of gamma-aminobutyric acid is known to cause convulsions in animals, and a convulsive disorder in human infants is due to vitamin B₆ deficiency.[2]

Pyridoxyl phosphate is also a cofactor of the enzyme kynureninase. The enzyme metabolizes kynurenine and 5-hydroxy kynurenine to anthranilic and 5-hydroxyanthranilic acids, the latter then going on to form niacin. In a state of vitamin B₆ deficiency, the kynurenines are changed instead by a transaminase to kynurenic and xanthurenic acids. A vitamin B₆ deficiency might lead to pellagra if the intake of niacin is marginal (see page 105).

Vitamin B₆ deficiency impairs the ability of the body to make glycine from glyoxalate and other substances, and the result is a considerable increase in the formation and urinary excretion of oxalate. This may be important in the formation of renal stones (page 178).

Pyridoxine is also needed for the synthesis of porphyrins from delta-aminolevulinic acid. In erythropoiesis, iron enters the

113

porphyrin molecule to form hemoglobin. Hence, a deficiency of vitamin B$_6$ leads to anemia of a peculiar kind, with very high serum and tissue iron levels.

Vitamin B$_6$ deficiency commonly causes neuropathy. Its exact mechanism is not, however, established, and the etiology of the condition in a given patient cannot be ascertained unless a good response to vitamin B$_6$ therapy has occurred. In addition, vitamin B$_6$ deficiency causes scaly skin changes, stomatitis, cheilosis, and perhaps depression of immune responses. The manifestations are all worsened by a high protein intake.

Sauerblich et al.[3] have given us a marvelously detailed, yet concise, discussion of the methods used to evaluate the vitamin B$_6$ status in human subjects. Blood levels and urine levels of vitamin B$_6$, or the urinary excretion of a metabolic pyridoxic acid, have all been used. Xanthurenic acid excretion after a tryptophan load has also been used. All these methods do not necessarily give comparable measurements.[3] Glutamic-oxalic transaminase (GOT) and glutamic-pyruvic transaminase levels in plasma, red blood cells, and leukocytes all fall in pyridoxine deficiency. The plasma levels are so low normally that these measurements are not useful in clinical studies. However, erythrocyte levels are apparently not suitable either for this purpose.[4] Laboratory evidence of deficiency, whatever methods may be used, may be present in patients with no evidence of clinical deficiency.

Vitamin B$_6$—like some other B-complex vitamins—is not stored in the human body to any great extent. Nevertheless, deficiencies owing purely to deficient intake are rare in normal persons, except infants. Even here the evidence suggests that at least some of the infants who develop the convulsions caused by B$_6$ deficiency have a congenitally increased need for the vitamin.

The situation in pregnancy and in the newborn is complicated. In the first place it must be recognized that a deficiency of the vitamin is common in pregnancy, usually manifesting itself by the symptoms of neuropathy, e.g. numbness and tingling of the extremities commonly encountered. A considerable literature now accumulated shows that estrogen interferes with the actions of the vitamin, and of course, estrogen production is very high in pregnancy. There has been some theoretical discussion about the possibility that B_6 deficiency might be responsible for psychosis in pregnancy in some cases. I know of no solid evidence in support of this view, but there is no harm in such cases in trying the vitamin in doses of 1.0 gram daily for a week or so. The recommended daily intake of 2.5 mg is not adequate for pregnant women.[5, 6] Even 10 mg per day given as a supplement may not be enough to keep the blood level normal.[5] A dose of 4.0 mg per day has been recommended as a routine.[6] Newborn babies whose mothers have low serum vitamin B_6 levels also show low levels.[5] The precise significance of the quantitative findings is difficult to state since newborn babies always have higher levels than do their mothers.[7] In the most recent studies, lactating mothers who took less than 2.5 mg per day of the vitamin produced milk low in B_6 content. However, increasing the intake much above 2.5 mg per day did not increase the milk concentration above that achieved with the 2.5 mg intake.[8] Nevertheless, it appears that whereas considerably more than 2.5 mg per day is needed by pregnant women, and presumedly by women postpartum, the data show that the amount of the vitamin they can give their nursing children in their milk cannot be increased by the mothers taking more than 2.5 mg per day. When compared to pregnant women, users of oral contraceptive pills may show even more marked deficiency of the vitamin.[4, 9, 10] Approximately 20 percent of women who take the pill have low serum levels of pyridoxal phosphate. The values are especially likely to be low in the age group twenty to thirty-four. In some, the levels rise again after some months. In some of the subjects studied,[4] the tryptophan-loading test revealed a deficiency of vitamin B_6 more often than did using serum pyridoxal levels below an arbitrary value of 5 mg per 100 ml. Brown et al.[11] used blood levels and concluded that the deficiency was likely to be common only when the diet was not adequate. However, when the tryptophan-loading test was used, a dose of 20 mg of vitamin B_6 a day was needed to counteract the effects of the estrogen in the contraceptive pills.[12] These deficiencies of vitamin B^6 are presumably responsible for the numbness, tingling, and other evidences of peripheral neuropathy encountered in pregnant women and in women taking oral contraceptives.

Another evidence of vitamin B₆ deficiency is anemia. Anemia occurs in pregnancy, especially in pre-eclampsia, and it may also occur in women who use oral contraceptives. In one study,[4] giving vitamin B₆ not only cured the anemia but raised the red blood cell counts considerably in nonpregnant women not taking estrogen. This phenomenon needs verification.

Still another change seen during pregnancy and in users of oral contraceptive pills is the development of mild diabetes mellitus. When this is studied in oral contraceptive users, the condition is found to be accompanied by a high serum insulin level.[13] The abnormal glucose tolerance induced by vitamin B₆ deficiency in the oral contraceptive users was reported reversed by giving the vitamin.[13]

Other side-effects of oral contraceptives, the acne and the skin pigmentation, are not relieved by vitamin B₆. In some cases the mental depression seems to be.

The vitamin B₆ deficiency of oral contraceptive use resembles that seen in pregnancy. Aside from this phenomenon, the occurrence of pyridoxine deficiency in adults is most commonly owing to the effects of medication. An excellent review by Roe[14] discusses the medications that cause the deficiency, viz., the hydrazines (isoniazide, iproniazide, marplan, nardil and niamid, and also hydralizine, l-dopa, and penicillamine).

Age seems to be a factor also. The serum level falls with advancing age, but even in some younger men, not economically deprived, low levels are sometimes found. With age there is an average decrease in the serum level of 7.3 percent per decade.[15]

Gastrointestinal disease also seems to be a factor. In one group of patients studied because they had dyspepsia, approximately 85 percent with gastric lesions had low serum pyridoxal levels. Some dyspeptic patients with no visible lesions also had low levels.[16] Perhaps their symptoms made them restrict their diets unwisely.

Special situations are created by alcoholism. In malnourished alcoholics the B₆ levels in both the serum and the cerebrospinal fluid are low, more so in those with evidence of brain damage.[17] The B₆ nutritional status is a highly complicated matter in alcoholics.

Alcoholics with liver disease absorb vitamin B$_6$ poorly from food.[18] This appears to be the result of the inability of these patients to break down the pyridoxal phosphate of food into pyridoxine so that it can be absorbed. Moreover, when a drink of alcohol is taken, some of the vitamin B$_6$ present in the liver leaves it.[19, 20] In addition, the common finding of low plasma pyridoxal phosphate levels in alcoholic patients without liver or hematologic abnormalities appears to be due to the excessive activity of a red blood cell phosphatase that hydrolyzes the vitamin.[21] This effect seems to be due to the acetaldehyde formed from alcohol and would seem to negate the effects of a good diet if one were taken.

It is remarkable how few studies of vitamin B$_6$ status have been made in nongastrointestinal disease. Several studies have been made in rheumatoid arthritis.[22] A majority of patients have low serum values, but giving 50 mg per day for months does not improve the syndrome, although the blood levels become normal or higher.

Uremia also causes vitamin B$_6$ deficiency.[23] This has interested many authors because many of the manifestations of uremia resemble those of vitamin B$_6$ deficiency. As a result of the B$_6$ deficiency the red blood cell glutamic-oxalic transaminase is low in uremia. Incubating the cells with pyridoxal phosphate has been found to stimulate the GOT in the cells of uremic patients, but not if the patients had been dialyzed. The clinical significance of the latter finding is not evident. It would be interesting to know whether some of the discomforts of uremia can be controlled with vitamin B$_6$.

Another condition that, in the eyes of some, resembles vitamin B$_6$ deficiency as regards metabolic changes, is Down's syndrome.[24] In this disease the concentration of the pyridoxal phosphate is low in the platelets and polymorphonuclear leukocytes, apparently because of an increase in the turnover rate.

A state of severe immunodepression is produced in animals when vitamin B$_6$ deficiency is induced.[25] Whether this fact is applicable in human medicine is not known, but it certainly should be studied.

RECOMMENDATIONS

Vitamin B_6 has little toxicity. Doses as large as 1,000 mg daily have been given without ill effect.

Pregnant women should receive 10 to 20 mg per day. Women taking oral contraceptives, likewise.

Alcoholics should take 10 to 100 mg a day if seemingly well and more if not.

Pyridoxine is without effect unless it reaches the body cells as the phosphate. Whether all the vitamin given by mouth reaches the cells in this form when body metabolism is distorted is not known. Hence, in these states even larger amounts might be tried.

For a discussion of the use of the vitamin in the prevention of oxalate nephrolithiasis, see page 178.

REFERENCES

1. Williams, M. A.: Present knowledge of vitamin B_6. In *Present Knowledge of Nutrition.* New York, The Nutrition Foundation, 1967, p. 66.
2. Coursin, D. B.: Vitamin B_6 and brain function in animals and man. *Ann NY Acad Sci, 166*:7, 1969.
3. Sauerblich, H. E., Canham, J. E., Baker, E. M., Raica, N., Jr., and Herman, Y. F.: Biochemical assessment of the nutritional status of vitamin B_6 in the human. *Am J Clin Nutr, 25*:629, 1972.
4. Shane, B. and Contractor, S. F.: Assessment of vitamin B_6 status. Studies on pregnant women and oral contraceptive users. *Am J Clin Nutr, 28*:739, 1975.
5. Cleary, R. E., Lumeng, L., and Li, T.-K.: Material and fetal plasma levels of pyridoxal phosphate at term. Adequacy of vitamin B_6 supplementation during pregnancy. *Am J Obstet Gynecol, 121*:25, 1975.
6. Lumeng, L., Cleary, R. E., Wagner, R., Yu, P.-L., and Li, T.-K.: Adequacy of vitamin B_6 supplementation during pregnancy: a prospective study. *Am J Clin Nutr, 29*:1376, 1976.
7. Bamji, M. S.: Enzymic evaluation of thiamine, riboflavin and pyridoxine status of parturient women and their newborn infants. *Br J Nutr, 35*:259, 1976.
8. West, K. D. and Kirksey, A.: Influence of vitamin B_6 intake on the content of the vitamin in human milk. *Am J Clin Nutr, 29*:961, 1976.

9. Lumeng, L., Cleary, R. E., and Li, T.-K.: Effect of oral contraceptives on the plasma concentration of pyridoxal phosphate. *Am J Clin Nutr*, 27:326, 1974.

10. Rose, D. P., Leklem, J. E., Brown, R. R., and Potera, C.: Effect of oral contraceptives and vitamin B_6 supplements on alanine and glycine metabolism. *Am J Clin Nutr*, 29:956, 1976.

11. Brown, R. R., Rose, D. P., Leklem, J. E., Linksweler, H. M., and Arend, R. A.: Urinary 4-pyridoxic acid, plasma pyridoxal phosphate, and erythrocyte aminotransferase levels in oral contraceptive users receiving controlled intakes in B_6. *Am J Clin Nutr*, 28:10, 1975.

12. Leklem, J. E., Brown, R. R., Rose, D. P., Linkswiler, H. M., and Arend, R. A.: Metabolism of tryptophan and niacin in oral contraceptive users receiving controlled intakes of vitamin B_6. *Am J Clin Nutr*, 28:146, 1975.

13. Rose, D. P., Leklem, J. E., Brown, R. R., and Linkswiler, H. M.: Effect of oral contraceptives and vitamin B_6 deficiency in carbohydrate metabolism. *Am J Clin Nutr*, 28:872, 1975.

14. Roe, D. A.: Drug-induced deficiency of B-vitamins. *NY State Med J*, 71:2770, 1971.

15. Rose, C. S., Gyorgy, P., Butler, M., Andres, R., Norris, A. H., Shock, N. W., Tobin, J., Brin, M., and Spiegel, H.: Age differences in vitamin B_6 status of 617 men. *Am J Clin Nutr*, 29:847, 1976.

16. Sanderson, C. R. and Davis, R. E.: Serum pyridoxal in patients with gastric pathology. *Gut*, 17:371, 1976.

17. Dastur, D. K., Santhadevi, N., Quadros, E. V., Avari, F. C. R., Wadia, N. H., Desai, M. M., and Bharucha, E. P.: The B-vitamins in malnutrition with alcoholism. *Br J Nutr*, 36:143, 1976.

18. Baker, H., Frank, O., Zetterman, R. K., Rajan, K. S., ten Hove, W., and Leevy, C. M.: Inability of alcoholics with liver disease to use food as a source of folates, thiamine, and vitamin B_6. *Am J Clin Nutr*, 28:1377, 1975.

19. Sorrell, M. F., Baker, H., Barak, A. J., and Frank, O.: Release by ethanol of vitamins into rat liver perfusate. *Am J Clin Nutr*, 27:743, 1974.

20. Frank, O., Linsada-Opper, A., Sorrell, M. F., Zetterman, R., and Baker, O.: Effects of a single intoxicating dose of ethanol on the vitamin profile of organelles in rat liver and brain. *J Nutr*, 106:606, 1976.

21. Lumeng, L. and Li, T.-K.: Vitamin B_6 metabolism in chronic alcohol abuse. *J Clin Invest*, 53:693, 1974.

22. Schumacher, H. R., Bernhart, F. W., and Gyorgy, P.: Vitamin B_6 levels in rheumatoid arthritis: effect of treatment. *Am J Clin Nutr*, 28:1200, 1975.

23. Sone, W. J., Warnock, L. G., and Wagner, C.: Vitamin B_6 deficiency in uremia. *Am J Clin Nutr*, 28:950, 1975.

24. Mahuren, J. D. and Coburn, S. P.: Pyridoxal phosphate in lymphocytes, polymorphonuclear leukocytes, and platelets in Down's syndrome. *Am J Clin Nutr, 27*:521, 1974.

25. Robson, L. C. and Schwartz, M. R.: Vitamin B$_6$ deficiency and the lymphoid system. I. Effects on cellular immunity and in vitro incorporation of ^{3}H-uridine by small lymphocytes. *Cell Immunol, 16*:135, 1975.

PANTOTHENIC ACID

As its name indicates, pantothenic acid seems to be universally present in living things, including living things destined to become part of the human diet. Hence, the likelihood of a deficiency of this substance occurring at all, and of being responsible for disease, seems remote. Even in severely malnourished alcoholic patients, the serum pantothenic acid level is only occasionally found to be low.[1] Only with difficulty can a deficiency state be induced in normal persons.[2] Nevertheless, in one study, teenage girls managed to take a diet deficient in the vitamin and, in some cases, to develop low serum concentrations of it.[3] Those girls who added becoming pregnant to these aberrations showed very low serum values which they maintained for some weeks postpartum. The infants' serum levels, although higher than their mothers', were still low. The authors of these studies recommend supplements of 10 to 15 mg per day in such cases.

The serum levels in vegetarians are much higher than those who take an ordinary diet.[4] In normal persons the serum level falls with age.[5] Few studies have been made in disease, and only chronic arthritis has been reported to be associated with low serum values.[4]

What we know about the clinical manifestations of pantothenic acid deficiency comes from the papers of Bean and Hodges and their co-workers.[2] The manifestations consist largely of a personality disorder in which irritability, unwillingness to get out of bed, restlessness, and quarrelsomeness, together with alternate periods of insomnia and somnolence occur. Fatigability, loss of drive, and sudden episodes of sweating are common. Epigastric burning, regurgitation, noisy intestines, and occasional diarrhea are the main somatic symptoms. Staggering gait and other evidences of incoordination may develop. There is nothing specific as regards physical or routine laboratory findings that might be helpful in making a diagnosis.

Actually, pantothenic acid by itself is physiologically inert. It must be changed into coenzyme A if it is to have any function. However, coenzyme A is involved in so many biochemical processes that it is impossible to conceive that its deficiency could cause any one type of clinical disorder. The only deficiency of coenzyme A despite adequate pantothenic acid nutrition that is known is purely a local phenomenon. In granulomatous or ulcerative colitis the diseased areas are unable to transform pantothenic acid into coenzyme A, although normal tissues in the same person can do so.[6] Whether this is cause or effect in this disease, and whether the biochemical abnormality affects in any way the cause of the illness is unknown. It is, however, worthy of note that when pigs are given a diet deficient in pantothenic acid, they develop ulcerative colitis. Nevertheless, there seems to be no reason to expect pantothenic acid to be therapeutic in human colitis.

RECOMMENDATIONS

In view of the widespread practice of cooking vegetables improperly, a daily supplement of perhaps 5 mg of pantothenic acid might be in order for careless eaters. In pregnancy this should be increased severalfold.

REFERENCES

1. Daster, D. K., Santhadevi, N., Quadros, E. V., Avari, F. C. R., Wadia, N. H., Desai, M. M., and Bharucha, E. P.: The B-vitamins in malnutrition with alcoholism. *Br J Nutr, 36*:143, 1976.
2. Hodges, R. E., Ohlson, M. A., and Bean, W. B.: Pantothenic acid deficiency in man. *J Clin Invest, 37*:1642, 1958.
3. Cohenour, S. H. and Calloway, D. H.: Blood, urine, and dietary pantothenic acid levels of pregnant teenagers. *Am J Clin Nutr, 25*:512, 1972.
4. Barton-Wright, E. C. and Elliott, W. A.: The pantothenic acid metabolism of rheumatoid arthritis. *Lancet, 2*:862, 1963.
5. Ishiguro, K., Kobayashi, S., and Kaneta, S.: Pantothenic acid content of human blood. *Tohoku J Exp Med, 74*:65, 1961.
6. Ellestad-Sayed, J. J., Nelson, R. A., Adson, M. A., Palmer, W. M., and Soule, E. H.: Pantothenic acid, coenzyme A, and human chronic ulcerative and granulomatous colitis. *Am J Clin Nutr, 29*:1333, 1976.

CYANOCOBALAMIN – VITAMIN B_{12}

VITAMIN B_{12} HAS BEEN recognized as a food factor for half a century, although its chemical identity has been known for a much shorter time. Some of its clinical features, i.e. macrocytosis, polynucleated leukocytes, and mental changes, do not in themselves distinguish vitamin B_{12} deficiency from folate deficiency. The achylia gastrica and neuropathy that are found regularly in primary pernicious anemia do help to distinguish this condition from folate deficiency. However, secondary B_{12} deficiency may occur without achylia gastrica. Vitamin B_{12} deficiency, like folate deficiency, causes a macrocytic bone-marrow picture, and this bone-marrow pattern may exist even in the absence of anemia. However, a deficiency of either vitamin B_{12} or folate (or both) may be recognized by low serum values for these substances even when the bone marrow appears normal.[1] Although low serum vitamin B_{12} levels are useful in diagnosis, in the last analysis only the absence of an intrinsic factor in gastric juice or the response to injections of adequate amounts of the vitamin can be considered conclusive. However, the latter conclusion is weakened by the fact that some patients with severe febrile illnesses who have vitamin B_{12} deficiency may fail to respond to the administered vitamin until the infection is controlled. Although the role of vitamin B_{12} in hematopoiesis has been most emphasized in clinical practice, the vitamin is important in maintaining the function of nerve tissue, as evidenced by the neuropathy and the mental changes associated with deficiency. The mental changes—depression, apathy, confusion, and even delusional and hallucinatory manifestations—are especially interesting because they may improve markedly after injection of the vitamin even before the first hematologic response in the form of reticulocytosis appears.

Patients with pernicious anemia of the primary type are likely to have a disorder of platelet function. Thrombocytopenia and prolonged bleeding time are common in them. Some exhibit abnormalities of platelet function,[2] consisting in deficient aggregation on stimulation, absent agglutination, and prolonged stypven time, the last indicating a deficient release of the factor that initiates clotting. During treatment with vitamin B_{12}, some of these low measurements became supernormal. This perhaps accounts for the thrombosis that sometimes accompanies treatment.

The biochemical role of vitamin B_{12} is not definitely established, although the vitamin seems to have something to do with nucleic acid synthesis. The increased urinary excretion of methylmalonic acid that occurs in vitamin B_{12} deficiency is not understood.

The daily dietary requirement of vitamin B_{12} is usually under three micrograms a day, an amount easily obtained from meat. Liver and kidneys are especially rich in the vitamin. However, many other foods contain vitamin B_{12} or close derivatives of it.[3] Some of these derivatives are not as readily absorbed from the gastrointestinal tract as is cyanocobalamin, the compound usually referred to as vitamin B_{12}. Cyanocobalamin is absorbed in normal persons in amounts equal to 40 to 80 percent of what is ingested.[3] The ready availability of the vitamin makes the deficiency occur in only a few circumstances: (a) so-called "primary pernicious anemia" is due to a lack of formation in the upper gastrointestinal tract of the intrinsic factor needed for the absorption of the vitamin; (b) a similar picture occurs after gastrectomy; (c) vitamin B_{12} deficiency may occur purely on a dietary basis in vegetarians; (d) some malabsorption syndromes may cause a deficiency; (e) vitamin B_{12} deficiency, formerly considered rare in pregnancy, is now recognized as not uncommon.

The liver is widely recognized as the chief site of storage of vitamin B_{12}. A recent study defined the normal bone-marrow content of the vitamin[4] and showed that it is approximately only 2 percent of the serum value, and the ratio between the two is quite variable. Both are, of course, low in megaloblastic anemia due to vitamin B_{12} deficiency.

Vitamin B_{12} is needed for the release of folate from the body stores, and hence, the two deficiencies often occur together. A detailed study of the vitamin B_{12} deficiency of pregnancy shows that the deficiency is always associated with folate deficiency.[1] Some authors, however, believe that the B$_{12}$ deficiency of pregnancy is owing to malabsorption secondary to impaired folate absorption, an effect of excess estrogen (page 108). It is true that vitamin B$_{12}$ deficiency may so affect small intestine function as to impair the absorption of the vitamin itself. This may render the Schilling test inaccurate.[5] Halsted[6] has contributed an excellent discussion of the status of the small intestine in vitamin B$_{12}$ and folate deficiencies.

The occurrence of vitamin B$_{12}$ deficiency after total gastrectomy is too well known to require comment here. What is less well known is the abnormal vitamin B$_{12}$ status after *partial* gastrectomy. In this condition, the finding of a normal Schilling test, which employs crystalline vitamin B$_{12}$, may throw no light on a patient's ability to absorb B$_{12}$ from food.[7] Actually, anemia is a common late complication of partial gastrectomy. It is often today ascribed solely to iron deficiency (in contrast to the anemia of total gastrectomy, which is usually believed to be of the pernicious anemia type). However, evaluation of the anemia of partial gastrectomy may be misleading, because any tendency to macrocytosis due to B$_{12}$ or folate deficiency is often masked by the accompanying iron deficiency. Mahmud et al. have recently discussed this.[8] Their study was made on 107 men who had had a partial gastrectomy an average of eight years previously. Fifty percent of them were anemic, the anemia being more common after Billroth II than after Billroth I operations. Although the serum B$_{12}$ level was low in only 37 percent of the patients, 68 percent had low erythrocyte B$_{12}$ levels. This suggests that currently accepted standards of B$_{12}$ deficiency are inadequate. In the patients studied, iron deficiency was found to be as important as B$_{12}$ deficiency in the genesis of the anemia. Folate deficiency, which was somewhat less common, was usually combined with B$_{12}$ deficiency when present.

Vitamin B$_{12}$ deficiency may also occur in malabsorption syndromes.

The occurrence of vitamin B$_{12}$ in vegetarians has been reviewed by Armstrong et al.[9] Their studies were made on an affluent vegetarian group, in contrast to earlier studies on Asian vegetarians. Their subjects had high serum folate levels and no evidence of iron deficiency. However, B_{12} deficiency was common, the serum B_{12} level correlating directly with the amount of meat and eggs taken. When the serum B_{12} level was lower than 160 picograms per ml, the patients were found to have a macrocytic anemia, with decreased red blood and white cell counts. However, all but one of this group had no symptoms.

A number of drugs may interfere with the absorption of vitamin B_{12}.[10] These include colchicine, neomycin, para-amino-benzoic acid, and the antidiabetic diguanides. The last named are, perhaps, the most interesting because confusion may arise about whether the neurological changes in a patient taking one of them is diabetic neuropathy or vitamin B_{12} deficiency.[11]

Some alcoholic patients develop vitamin B_{12} deficiency. This is probably at least partially due to deficient intake but, on the other hand, the possible role of folate deficiency in depressing vitamin B_{12} absorption must be considered. Moreover, the presence of alcohol in the blood perfusing the liver causes a very large loss of stored vitamin B_{12} from the liver, and the vitamin cannot reenter the liver stores as long as alcohol is in the blood.[12] It is only the small normal requirement for this vitamin that prevents the more frequent occurrence of clinical evidence of a deficiency of it. In fact, in one study of malnourished alcoholics in India, a deficiency of vitamin B_{12} did not occur.[13]

The finding of very low serum vitamin B_{12} levels in patients on a regimen of repetitive dialysis is of interest. Some of these patients may exhibit signs of neuropathy, which can be reversed only by large parenteral doses of the vitamin.[14]

The question about what to treat comes up. Patients may have low serum B_{12} values with no recognizable symptoms. When neuropathy occurs, it is not likely to be overlooked, but anemia, if not severe, may occur without any manifestations whatsoever except for the characteristic yellowish pallor. Mental changes may occur, and their relation to the B_{12} deficiency may not be recognized.

Is vitamin B_{12} useful in patients who have neither clinical nor laboratory evidence of a deficiency? Some puzzling reports have appeared in the English literature. The last of them, typical of the entire group, except that it was carried out double-blind, reports that giving 5 mg of vitamin B_{12} by injection twice a week for two weeks greatly helped the symptom of fatigue in patients whose only complaint was that symptom.[15] It is impossible to find fault with this study except that the symptom of fatigue is notably difficult to evaluate. The vitamin B$_{12}$ was given in pharmacologic doses and not as a nutritional supplement.

RECOMMENDATIONS

Vitamin B$_{12}$ deficiency does not occur in persons who eat meat or eggs unless they have a deficiency of intrinsic factor, either inborn or secondary to total gastrectomy. Although mammalian liver and kidneys, especially the former, are rich in the vitamin, there is no need to make a special point of eating them. When vitamin B$_{12}$ deficiency does develop in association with inadequate intake, it is due to food faddism or omission of meat and eggs from the diet for religious reasons, or because pregnancy has decreased nutritional intake at the same time as it imposes increased needs for the vitamin. In all these circumstances the patients cannot, or will not, take appropriate food in adequate amounts and, hence, must receive the vitamin by injection. Where B$_{12}$ deficiency is secondary to some type of gastrointestinal dysfunction that impairs absorption or destroys the vitamin in the intestinal tract, the vitamin must also be given by injection.

REFERENCES

1. Lowenstein, L., Brunton, L., and Hsich, X.-S.: Nutritional anemia and megaloblastosis in pregnancy. *Can Med Assoc J*, *94*:636, 1966.
2. Levine, P. H.: A qualitative platelet defect in severe vitamin B$_{12}$ deficiency. Response, hyperresponse, and thrombosis after vitamin B$_{12}$ therapy. *Ann Intern Med*, 78:533, 1973.
3. Farquarson, J. and Adams, J. F.: The forms of vitamin B$_{12}$ in foods. *Br J Nutr*, *36*:127, 1976.
4. Trubowitz, S., Frank, O., and Baker, H.: Survey of vitamin B$_{12}$ and folate in the serum and marrow tissue of hospitalized patients. *Am J Clin Nutr*, *27*:580, 1974.
5. Carmel, R. and Herbert, V.: Correctable intestinal defect of vitamin B$_{12}$ absorption in pernicious anemia. *Ann Intern Med*, *67*:1201, 1967.
6. Halsted, C. H.: The small intestine in vitamin B$_{12}$ and folate deficiency. *Nutr Rev*, *33*:33, 1975.

7. Mahmud, K., Ripley, D., and Doscherholmen, A.: Vitamin B_{12} absorption tests. Their unreliability in postgastrectomy states. *JAMA*, *216*:1167, 1971.

8. Mahmud, K., Ripley, D., Swaim, W. R., and Doscherholmen, A.: Hematologic complications of partial gastrectomy. *Ann Surg*, *177*: 432, 1973.

9. Armstrong, B. K., Davis, R. E., Nicol, D. J., van Merwyk, A. J., and Larwood, C. J.: Hematological, vitamin B_{12}, and folate studies on Seventh Day Adventist vegetarians. *Am J Clin Nutr*, *27*:712, 1974.

10. Gaginella, T. S.: Drug-induced malabsorption. *Drug Therapy*, December, 1975.

11. Tomkin, G. H., Hadden, D. R., Weaver, J. A., and Montgomery, D. A. D.: Vitamin B_{12} status of patients on long-term metformin therapy. *Br Med J*, *2*:685, 1971.

12. Sorrell, M. F., Baker, H., Barak, A. J., and Frank, O.: Release by ethanol of vitamins into rat liver perfusates. *Am J Clin Nutr*, *27*:743, 1974.

13. Dastur, D. K., Santhadevi, N., Quadros, E. V., Avari, F. C. R., Wadia, N. H., Desai, M. M., and Bharucha, E. P.: The B-vitamins in malnutrition with alcoholism. *Br J Nutr*, *36*:143, 1976.

14. Rostand, S. G.: Vitamin B_{12} levels and nerve conduction velocities in patients undergoing maintenance hemodialysis. *Am J Clin Nutr*, *29*:691, 1976.

15. Ellis, F. R. and Nasser, S.: A pilot study of vitamin B_{12} in the treatment of tiredness. *Br J Nutr*, *30*:277, 1973.

FLAVONOIDS

T HE ROLE OF flavonoids in biochemical processes is both varied and extensive, to judge by the reported studies. Their role in human disease has remained unproven. A recent report indicates a possible place for some flavonoids in human clinical medicine.

It is known that the cataracts that occur in diabetes mellitus and in galactosemia develop owing to the action of an enzyme, aldose reductase. This enzyme accelerates the change of glucose and galactose to their respective polyols, sorbitol and galactitol. These polyols are present in the lens in diabetes (and in galactosemia) in very large amounts and, by acting osmotically, overhydrate the lens. Ultimately, cataracts develop. The enzyme is inhibited by flavonoids, and giving these compounds to diabetic animals has greatly delayed the development of cataracts in them.[1] Since these compounds are innocuous, they might be used in patients in doses of 1.0 gram per day.

REFERENCE

1. Varma, S. D., Mizuno, A., and Kinoshita, J. H.: Diabetic cataracts and flavonoids. *Science, 195*:205, 1977.

ASCORBIC ACID – VITAMIN C

A MOST INTERESTING aspect of the development of clinical knowledge about vitamin C is that the knowledge seems to be highly forgettable. Mariners during the fifteenth and sixteenth century explorations of America knew about preventing or curing scurvy by eating green vegetables. The American Indians knew about it before that. In the British navy, James Lind, who wrote in 1747, and James Cook, who wrote in 1772, are today given credit for discovering how to prevent scurvy. American Revolutionary armies nevertheless suffered from scurvy and were defeated by it rather than by opposing forces. Some British armies in the Crimean War and even in World War I had more scurvy than gunshot casualties. The explorers Shackleton and Scott, on a *scientific* expedition to the Antarctic in 1914, ignored what had been recorded about scurvy during the previous centuries and paid a high price for having forgotten the lessons of the past. Today the clinical studies of vitamin C losses in disease made a generation or two ago have been forgotten.

Ascorbic acid has aroused a great amount of controversy. This is owing to several factors: Its physiologic role is not adequately known; it is a vitamin for some species and not others; its actions are greatly influenced by stress. It is not possible to be certain about the daily requirement for man.

Chatterjee[1] has written an excellent account of the way in which the synthesis of ascorbic acid has evolved. Invertebrates and fish do not synthesize it and, hence, must be getting all they need from their food. Fish scurvy is a recognized disease. The amphibia and the reptiles make ascorbic acid in their kidneys. Mammals, with the exception of primates, the guinea pig, and the flying mammals, manufacture the ascorbic acid they require in their livers. The species that cannot manufacture vitamin C all lack the terminal enzyme l-gulonolactone oxidase. Baboons living wild get about 4 grams of ascorbic acid in their diet of

uncooked vegetation. It is not known whether they actually need this much. Consequently, data obtained on them cannot be used to estimate optimal human intakes, as some have presumed to do. Nevertheless, it is clear that 4 grams of ascorbic acid a day is not toxic to at least that primate.

Studies of the amounts of ascorbic acid in the tissues have been made. They show that the leukocyte ascorbic acid level may remain normal after the plasma level has fallen. However, the ascorbic acid levels of tissues may fall although the leukocyte concentration remains normal. Which, then, is the best guide to the status of the tissues—the plasma level or the leukocyte level? It is clear that the latter is a poor guide, and available evidence unfortunately indicates that the former is also. It appears that there is no laboratory test to diagnose accurately mild or moderate ascorbic acid deficiency or to evaluate treatment in severe deficiency of the vitamin. As will be discussed later, the passage of the vitamin from plasma to leukocytes may be inhibited, causing a reversal of the usual sequence in which plasma is depleted before the leukocytes are. Moreover, some tissues may build up a large store of ascorbic acid and then lose it, with no change in plasma ascorbic acid level. Thus, the human fetal brain has a very much larger amount of ascorbic acid than the adult.[2] This falls during fetal life, but even at birth the human infant's brain has at least three times as much as the adult's. The blood of the human infant at birth has at least four times more ascorbic acid than its mother's.[2] How the fetus is able to take so much ascorbic acid from its mother is not known. The phenomenon violates the known principles of diffusion of molecules similar to ascorbic acid. After birth the serum ascorbic acid level falls markedly during the first year of life[3] and probably thereafter.

Questions have arisen about the comparative availability for use in man of ascorbic acid manufactured synthetically, as compared to ascorbic acid extracted or concentrated (by means of chemical techniques) from food sources. Studies of the absorption from the intestinal tract of these two kinds of ascorbic acid have been made[4] and show no differences.

The recommended daily intake of vitamin C in man is a matter of controversy.[5] The "Recommended Daily Allowances" sound authoritative but are not. The most commonly used methods, i.e. to study the amount of the vitamin in the urine, the blood plasma, and the leukocytes, are not demonstrably valid. In fact, there is good reason to doubt their usefulness. A recent study used a different approach, i.e. the establishment in the guinea pig of the amount of the vitamin needed not to prevent overt scurvy but to prevent any changes at all as seen in the electron microscopic examination of the buccal mucous membrane.[6] The amount of vitamin C needed to prevent any change at all was approximately one hundred times greater than the amount needed merely to prevent overt scurvy. How much ascorbic acid do we then need? The answer is not easily established, because there are large variations in requirements caused by individual variations, by age, by sex hormones, and by a variety of stress factors.

The laboratory studies and literature reviews published by Loh and Wilson[7] are remarkable for their breadth and depth. There is a daily rhythm in the plasma and leukocyte ascorbic acid concentration, the values being highest at midnight and lowest at noon. A rise in blood leukocyte count is accompanied by a fall in leukocyte ascorbic acid concentration. Ascorbic acid taken by mouth becomes dehydroascorbic acid, and this is changed back to ascorbic acid by the red blood cells from which the vitamin diffuses into the plasma. The leukocytes take it from there, but the leukocytes may contain the vitamin even when the plasma concentration is zero. The leukocytes become saturated with the vitamin where the intake of it is 200 mg or more. Young women who are taking 500 mg a day show a sudden increase in urinary output on the fourteenth day of the menstrual cycle, corresponding to the peak excretion of luteinizing hormone (LH).[7]

The last half dozen years have seen the publication of a number of remarkable reports that resulted from collaborative studies by laboratories of the Department of Medicine, University of Iowa, and laboratories of the U.S. Army's Fitzsimmons General Hospital.[8-14] The studies used radioactively tagged ascorbic acid and followed the excretion of the tagged ascorbate and other substances. The reported observations add to our knowledge of the metabolism but they leave many questions unanswered and indeed raise some not previously recognized.

Normal men seem to contain a pool of 1500 mg of ascorbic acid. This is no ordinary pool, for it equilibrates slowly with the brain ascorbic acid. Much administered ascorbic acid does not enter this pool at all. Hence, the physiologic significance of this pool is ambiguous. At any rate, changes in its magnitude can be correlated more or less with physiologic and psychologic manifestations. At about the time the size of the pool, as calculated, has fallen by 60 percent, disabling psychologic symptoms appear. They comprise neurotic, hypochondriacal, and hysteric symptoms. Fatigue, lassitude, and depression are among the notable findings. Paranoia has also occurred (the control subjects were on a vitamin A deficient diet and developed no such symptoms). Measured psychomotor performance deteriorates somewhat later.

In the studies reported, as the daily intake of vitamin C was maintained at zero, the urine output of the vitamin fell, ultimately reaching zero. However, four as yet unidentified substances related to vitamin C continued to be found in the urine in substantial amounts. The blood and serum levels fell, but not to zero. Neither the blood or serum level nor the urine level indicated the size of the body pool.

When the body pool fell to approximately 300 mg, i.e. only 20 percent of normal, the signs of scurvy began to develop. However, the rate and sequence of appearance of the scorbutic symptoms varied greatly, even though all the subjects were maintained in the same milieu and on the same diet. The well-known scorbutic hemorrhages, perifollicular hyperkeratosis, and gum swelling were observed but, in addition, unexpected manifestations also developed. These were acne, joint pain and swelling, muscle pain, excessive small vessel vasoconstriction on exposure to cold or after intra-arterial infusion of norepinephrine, negative nitrogen balance, fall in plasma albumin leading to oliguria and to edema, neuropathy, increased sensitivity to the hypoglycemic effect of insulin, and unexpected increases in the urinary output of pyridoxine.

It should be noted that the subjects became ill long before

they exhibited scorbutic manifestations. During the studies several other things became evident. When one of the subjects developed an anxious depression not due to vitamin C deficiency, his urinary vitamin C output increased markedly. Also, when the intake of a salt mixture, made up chiefly of phosphates and iron together with lesser amounts of other salts, was decreased, the loss of ascorbic acid from the body pool also became accelerated.

Giving the subjects vitamin C restored their body pools and relieved their symptoms. However, on a fixed intake of the vitamin, two rates of repletion of the pool were observed—an early, fast rate and a later, slower one. As noted before, with large intakes some or most of the administered vitamin C failed to enter the pool. However, there are at least two other pools related to, but not the same as, the vitamin C pool. Hence, at present, attempts to do balance studies on ascorbic acid cannot be planned, much less carried out.

Although all the functions of vitamin C are not known, several have been adequately defined. A vast amount of experimental work, as well as many observations in human disease, have shown that vitamin C is required to maintain the integrity of the wall of small blood vessels. It is also essential to the manufacture of collagen. Its role in collagen formation depends largely on its function as an activator of the enzyme prolyl hydroxylase.[15] Since hydroxyproline is not only the essential but also the characteristic amino acid of collagen, the importance of the enzyme is obvious. The significance of this biochemical phenomenon was demonstrated neatly in man by Liakokas et al.[16] These authors studied urinary hydroxyproline excretion in children given corticosteroids. These steroids are known to inhibit collagen formation—in fact, this is one of the chief adverse effects of steroid medication. Associated with this is a large decrease in the output of hydroxyproline. The children's hydroxyproline output rose by more than 50 percent when 1.5 grams of vitamin C were given daily. This study showed not only that vitamin C accelerates the formation of hydroxyproline, the essential constituent of collagen, but afforded a therapeutic suggestion for the control of the poor wound healing, and perhaps also the osteoporosis, that limits the clinical use of corticosteroids.

Another enzyme that seems to be activated by ascorbic acid

is alcohol dehydrogenase, the liver enzyme that helps dispose of alcohol that reaches the liver in the blood.[17] In the study by Krasner et al.[17] the leukocyte ascorbic acid level and the liver alcohol dehydrogluconase activity were found to be parallel through a wide range of values. In addition, the rate of removal of administered alcohol from the blood stream was measured in normal persons before and again after a two-week period in which each received one gram of ascorbic acid daily. The rate of alcohol removal paralleled the leukocyte ascorbic acid level. Evidently alcoholic drinks made with citrus fruit juices may have some benefits.

Biochemists have long emphasized that ascorbic acid is an antioxidant in isolated subcellular biological systems. The significance of this property for clinical conditions has been ambiguous ever since its discovery. However, it now appears that the antioxidant property of vitamin C can be shown to be important in one clinical condition. A macrocytic anemia caused by folate deficiency can occur in scurvy.[18] During the period of lack of vitamin C, folate is oxidized abnormally to 10-formyl folate, which deprives the body of the normal tetrahydroformates that are responsible for the antianemic property of folate. This induced folate deficiency interferes with the incorporation of hemoglobin into the red blood cells.

Ascorbic acid is also important in iron metabolism. The absorption of iron from the intestinal tract depends on the dose of vitamin C given.[19] Women need more ascorbic acid than men to maintain normal hematopoiesis. Ascorbic acid is also important in maintaining iron stores and the transfer of iron from the blood stream to the liver, where it is stored as ferritin.[20]

Vitamin C metabolism is also affected by sex hormones. Plasma vitamin C levels fall during the course of pregnancy.[2] The menstrual cycle also affects ascorbic acid metabolism.[7] Estrogen lowers the ascorbic acid content of plasma and the blood lekuocytes and platelets.[21] This is not owing to an increase in the excretion of the vitamin and, hence, must be caused by some tissue changes.

Aspirin seriously impairs vitamin C effectiveness. Whether this is owing to the salicylate itself or to its chief metabolic product, orthohydroxyhippuric acid, is not known. This is im-

to ascertain because orthohydroxyhippuric acid is formed
,tress of almost any kind, even though no aspirin is taken.[22]
__, prevents the transfer of plasma vitamin C into leukocytes
and, presumably, other tissues, even though high plasma levels
are maintained.[23] In these circumstances there is a simultaneous
increase in urinary ascorbic acid output. Giving aspirin daily
for more than four days causes a fall in plasma and leukocyte
ascorbic acid levels almost to those found in scurvy.[23] A dose of
two aspirin tablets (600 mg) prevents the entry into the leukocytes of ascorbic acid in doses of up to 1 gram.[24] The interference
with blood platelet function caused by aspirin impairs blood
clotting and hemostasis.

The fact that aspirin interferes with ascorbic acid transfer
must have influenced the outcome of studies on colds, since many
persons with upper respiratory infections take aspirin. In addition,
the course and symptoms of the common cold are so variable
and ambiguous as to create wonder in the minds of some physicians
about why anyone would spend huge sums of money and use
huge amounts of time in trying to prove by clinical statistical
studies the efficacy of vitamin C in preventing colds, or at least
some of the symptoms. Nevertheless, these studies go on. Wilson,
Greene, and Loh have made an important contribution in this
dubious field because they made metabolic studies.[25] During a
cold, the plasma and leukocyte vitamin C levels fall markedly.
Giving single doses of 500 to 1000 mg did cause a rise in plasma
levels, but the leukocyte concentrations continued to fall, presumably because of the utilization of the vitamin C in other
tissues. Giving two grams of ascorbic acid to persons with
colds raised the plasma levels in both sexes, but only in women
did this dose raise the leukocyte concentration. The salivary
and lingual ascorbic acid levels also fall during a cold, more or
less parallel with the fall in leukocyte values. Presumably a dose
of 2 grams is adequate to restore tissue ascorbic acid status in
women, but more is apparently needed in men. It is worthy of
note that some of the clinical trials have indicated that female
patients with colds are more likely to benefit from the supplemental ascorbic acid than are male subjects. It is interesting that
D-isoascorbic acid, although it has little antiscurvy activity,

appears to be more effective than ascorbic acid itself in 1 gram doses.[26]

Whatever one may think about the importance of vitamin C in the prevention or treatment of cold symptoms, the fact remains that metabolic studies on the cold call attention to and reinforce the results of studies in stress.

There are a great many studies in animals, mostly rodents, that show that supplemental vitamin C protects against effects of life-threatening factors such as extreme cold and the injection of bacterial toxins or histamine. In these experiments the added ascorbic acid amounts to ten to one hundred times the amounts usually fed to the animals. Experiments of this sort obviously cannot be carried out in man, nor can the data of the extreme states produced in the animals be applied to clinical conditions in man. As Baker's review[27] shows, there are surprisingly few data on stress in man. One related study is of great interest. It has been shown that concentrations of ascorbic acid many times greater than that of blood but equal to that of some tissues greatly stimulates leukocyte activity.[28]*

The effect of heat and humidity on vitamin C output has been studied. Heat itself has no effect on urinary output and little on sweat concentration of the vitamin. There is little excreted in sweat.[29] However, humidity plus heat doubles the urinary output.[30] The serum ascorbic acid level is low in Europeans living in the tropics.[31]

In one study cigarette smokers had lower serum vitamin C levels than nonsmokers despite adequate intakes of the vitamin.[32] Those who smoked twenty or more cigarettes showed a 40 percent reduction. Cigarette smoke causes the formation of free-radicals in the body,[33] and they are known to be capable of oxidizing ascorbic acid. However, in another study[34] no great change was found, perhaps because few cigarettes were smoked.

---

* Similar findings have been reported in relation to steroid therapy. Corticosteroids are known to inhibit leukocytic function. This disorder is reversed by giving 2.0 gm. of ascorbic acid over a twelve-hour period, according to Chretien, J. H. and Garagusi, V. F. (Correction of corticosteroid-induced defects of polymorphonuclear neutrophil function by ascorbic acid. *J Reticuloendothel Soc,* 14:280, 1973.)

As was noted previously, estrogen, as in oral contraceptive pills, lowers the plasma ascorbic acid level.[21] A similar fall occurs in pregnancy.[35] The effects of the fall in plasma ascorbic acid that occurs during pregnancy are not completely known. It is possible that the ascorbic acid deficiency contributes to folate deficiency (see page 136). There is also a report that pregnant women who take supplementary ascorbic acid bear fewer children with birth defects than women who do not.[35]

Little work has been done on the role of ascorbic acid deficiency in human disease. Goldsmith[36] reviewed earlier literature and concluded that a wide variety of disease states increased the vitamin C requirement. A little later Scrimshaw[37] reviewed the effects of stress on nutrition and provided a list of references that describe the fall in serum ascorbic acid level that occurs in a wide variety of febrile illnesses. Kyhos et al.[38] made observations on a group of patients with a variety of chronic diseases and with a history suggestive of deficient intake of vitamin C. Most of them had very low serum—in some cases, zero. Urinary excretion was also low. Giving as much as 1.5 grams of the vitamin at a time in some cases produced no increase in urinary output, although the plasma level rose to normal. The amount of vitamin needed to bring the amount excreted in the urine to a constant normal level ("saturation" level) was between 1.5 and 2.8 grams. When depleted, the patients had no clinical evidence of this state except perhaps for what might have been nonspecific gum changes.

Levenson et al.[39] studied six persons who had received serious injuries; some had developed consequent to hemorrhage and infection. They were well nourished before the accidents. The serum ascorbic acid levels were very low and little was put out in the urine. Giving the vitamin in 1.0 gram doses resulted in an increased urinary output for some days. Evidently the trauma had increased the utilization of the vitamin greatly. However, when depleted, the patients had no clinical signs of scurvy.

Patients with peptic ulcers usually have laboratory evidence of vitamin C depletion.[40] This is true in uncomplicated ulcer disease, owing presumably to the fact that cow's milk, a main article of diet, contains little of the vitamin, and fruits and green vegetables are likely to be excluded from the diet. The deficiency may favor the occurrence of hemorrhage. Patients studied after operations for ulcer may have even more serious depletion. A similar depletion is also found in regional enteritis[40] and may interfere with healing.

Interesting observations on what is usually considered non-physical stress have also been made. Thus Maas et al.[41] studied anxious and nonanxious patients with either schizophrenia or with neurosis or personality disorders. The patients had no detectable physical illnesses and had not had psychoactive drugs. The plasma ascorbic acid levels were low in almost all cases. Milner reviewed this and subsequent work in his report.[42] He carried out a double-blind controlled study of the effects of 1 gram of ascorbic acid daily for three weeks in twenty patients, comparing the results in twenty others who received a placebo. Sixteen of the total of forty had mild skin changes of vitamin C deficiency, and all forty had low urine outputs of the vitamin before the experiment. Those who received the vitamin took an average of six days to reach a plateau of excretion (which was 800 mg per day). The Minnesota Multiphasic Personality Inventory (MMPI) rating scale showed improvement (p < .01) in the treated group and insignificant improvement in the placebo group. Particularly striking was the improvement in the depression factor in the MMPI measurements. In the patients studied, hospitalized an average of 17.7 years and with a mean age of 52.6 years, any improvement is astonishing.

A number of authors, noting the poor intake of foods containing vitamin C in the aged, have tried to relate the non-specific symptoms of malnutrition to ascorbic acid deficiency. Bermond[43] found a good correlation between the plasma ascorbic acid level and the frequency of such symptoms. These data are not clinically convincing because of the inadequacy of the plasma vitamin C level to describe the state of ascorbic acid nutrition and the vagueness of nonspecific symptoms of malnutrition. On the other hand, the data cannot be ignored. Bermond also found a linear inverse relation between age and plasma ascorbic acid level.

A number of other phenomena have been studied and, although the results are interesting, they cannot yet be evaluated as regards human disease. Thus, reports that ascorbic acid retards cancer-

cell growth and prevents diet-induced atherosclerosis in animals
have no evident application to man. Similarly, although scorbutic
animals seem to have some type of diabetes mellitus, giving 1.0
to 2.0 grams of ascorbic acid intravenously to normal, obese, or
diabetic patients was found to have no discernible effect on
glucose metabolism.[44]

There is, of course, vitamin C in all plant foods. However,
much is lost in cooking, but those who eat raw vegetables avoid
this loss. Citrus fruits and tomatoes contain appreciable amounts.
Milk has very little. Patients with ulcers who live on milk and
a low vegetable diet need added vitamin C, perhaps 500 mg or
more, in addition to whatever else they may need for other
reasons. Rheumatoid arthritis requires special comment. The
practice of giving large amounts of aspirin in one form or another
is a well-established one in medicine. This prevents the passage
of vitamin C from the plasma to the tissues, and hence, measuring
plasma or leukocyte levels to assess possible deficiencies is useless.
It is probable that patients with this disease would benefit from
energetic vitamin C therapy.

Reported work shows that vitamin C deficiency, even when
it has reached scorbutic levels, can be cured in a small group
of persons with 10 mg per day of vitamin C. Hence, we may
conclude that 10 mg per day is the daily requirement for preventing scurvy in at least some healthy, nonsmoking men in an
equable climate, free from serious emotional upset and not
suffering from trauma or severe infection. This minimal figure
applies not only to the cure—and prevention—of scurvy in such
persons, but also to the prevention of the other symptoms that
may occur without the appearance of overt manifestations of
scurvy. This minimal figure does not, however, allow for the
large variations in biochemical makeup that a normal population
exhibits. There are undoubtedly some normal persons who need
five or ten times the minimal amounts stated here.

The possibility has been raised that taking large amounts of
ascorbic acid might be harmful. It is true that one of the
metabolites of vitamin C is oxalate, and this substance is known
to give rise under some circumstances to kidney stones when
it is excreted in the urine. However, the urinary excretion of

oxalic acid increases only when the dose of ascorbic acid is over four grams per day.[45, 46] If the urine is markedly acid as the oxalate is excreted, there is a possibility that kidney stones will form. However, this occurrence has never been observed.[47] Nevertheless, it must be remembered that oxalate excretion is also increased by some vitamin deficiencies (page 176).

The fact that 4.0 grams of ascorbic acid doubles the urine output of uric acid is interesting but does not seem therapeutically useful. In the reported studies, the daily ingestion of 8.0 grams for three to seven days led to a fall in serum uric acid level of 1.2 to 3.1 mg per 100 ml.[48] The possibility of creating uric acid kidney stones exists, but the doses used in the study are far outside the range of clinical custom.

RECOMMENDATIONS

A review of the soundest literature available, as discussed above, permits the following conservative estimates to be formulated to meet the added needs induced by the vicissitudes of daily life among normal people. The available evidence suggests the following table of minimal figures for the daily intake of vitamin C.

	Men	*Women*
Basal	10 mg	20 mg
Humid climate	add 20	add 20
Cigarette smoking	add 20	add 20
Contraceptive pill	—	200
Pregnancy	—	300
Aspirin	200	200
Colds	add 500	add 200
Strong emotion	add 1000	add 1000
Trauma; severe infection	add 1000	add 1000
Heavy drinking	add 1000	add 1000

The amount that drug addicts should take cannot be estimated from the data at hand but is also probably large. In addition, ascorbic acid is important with respect to specific diseases as discussed above and for improving the absorption of iron in anemic people, who should receive it in gram doses.

REFERENCES

1. Chatterjee, I. B.: Evolution and the biosynthesis of ascorbic acid. *Science, 182*:1272, 1974.
2. Adlard, B. P. F., De Souza, S. W., and Moon, S.: Ascorbic acid in the fetal human brain. *Arch Dis Child, 49*:278, 1974.
3. Vobecky, J. S., Vobecky, J., Shapcott, D., and Blanchard, R.: Vitamin E and C levels in infants during the first year of life. *Am J Clin Nutr, 29*:766, 1976.
4. Nelson, E. W., Streiff, R. R., and Cerdoc, J. J.: Comparative bioavailability of folate and vitamin C from a synthetic and a natural source. *Am J Clin Nutr, 28*:1014, 1975.
5. Yew, M. L. S.: Recommended daily allowances for vitamin C. *Proc Natl Acad Sci USA, 70*:965, 1973.
6. Thaete, L. G., and Grim, J. W.: Fine structural effects of 1-ascorbic acid on buccal epithelium. *Am J Clin Nutr, 27*:719, 1974.
7. Loh, H. S., Odumasu, A., and Wilson, C. W. M.: Factors influencing the metabolic availability of ascorbic acid. 1. The effect of sex. *Clin Pharmacol Ther, 16*:390, 1974.
8. Hodges, R. E., Baker, E. M., Hood, J., Sauerblich, H. E., and March, S. C.: Experimental scurvy in man. *Am J Clin Nutr, 22*:535, 1969.
9. Hood, J. and Hodges, R. E.: Ocular lesions in scurvy. *Am J Clin Nutr, 22*:559, 1969.
10. Baker, E. M., Hodges, R. E., Hood, J., Sauerblich, H. E., and March, S. C.: Metabolism of ascorbic-1-^{14}C acid in experimental human scurvy. *Am J Clin Nutr, 22*:549, 1969.
11. Hodges, R. E., Hood, J., Canham, J. E., Sauerblich, H. E., and Baker, E. M.: Clinical manifestations of ascorbic acid deficiency in man. *Am J Clin Nutr, 24*:432, 1971.
12. Baker, E. M., Hodges, R. E., Hood, J., Sauerblich, H. E., March, S. C., and Canham, J. E.: Metabolism of ^{14}C and ^{3}H-labeled 1-ascorbic acid in human scurvy. *Am J Clin Nutr, 24*:444, 1971.
13. Krisman, R. A. and Hood, J.: Some behavioral aspects of ascorbic acid deficiency. *Am J Clin Nutr, 24*:455, 1971.
14. Baker, E. M., Kennedy, J. E., Tolbert, L. M., and Canham, J. E.: Excretion and body pool size of ascorbate sulphate and other ascorbate derivatives in man. *Fed Proc, 31*:704, 1972.
15. Stassen, F. L. H., Cardinale, G. J., and Udenfriend, S.: *Proc Natl Acad Sci USA, 70*:1090, 1973.
16. Liakokas, D., Ikhos, D. G., Vlachos, P., Ntalles, K., and Coulouris, C.: Effect of ascorbic acid on urinary hydroxyproline of children receiving corticosteroids. *Arch Dis Child, 49*:400, 1974.
17. Krasner, N., Dow, J., Moore, M. R., and Goldberg, A.: Ascorbic acid saturation and ethanol metabolism. *Lancet, 2*:693, 1974.
18. Stokes, P. L., Melikian, V., Leeming, R. L., Portman-Graham, H.,

Blair, J. A., and Cooke, W. T.: Folate metabolism in scurvy. *Am J Clin Nutr*, 28:126, 1975.

19. Nicholson, J. T. L. and Chernock, F. W.: Incubation studies of the human small intestine. An improved technique for the study of absorption and its application to ascorbic acid. *J Clin Invest*, 21:505, 1942.

20. Mazur, A.: Role of ascorbic acid in the incorporation of plasma iron into ferritin. *Ann NY Acad Sci*, 92:223, 1961.

21. Rivers, J. M.: Oral contraceptives and ascorbic acid. *Am J Clin Nutr*, 28:550, 1975.

22. Altshule, M. D. and Hegedus, Z. L.: Orthohydroxyhippuric (salicyluric) acid—its physiologic and clinical significance. *Clin Pharmacol Ther*, 15:111, 1974.

23. Loh, H. S., Walters, K., and Wilson, C. W. M.: The effects of aspirin on the metabolic availability of ascorbic acid in human beings. *J Clin Pharmacol*, 13:480, 1973.

24. Loh, H. S. and Wilson, C. W. M.: The interactions of aspirin and ascorbic acid in normal man. *J Clin Pharmacol*, 15:36, 1975.

25. Wilson, C. W. M., Greene, M., and Loh, H. S.: The metabolism of supplementary vitamin C during the common cold. *J Clin Pharmacol*, 16:19, 1976.

26. Clegg, K. M. and MacDonald, J. M.: 1-Ascorbic acid and D-isoascorbic acid in a common cold survey. *Am J Clin Nutr*, 28:973, 1975.

27. Baker, E. M.: Vitamin C requirements in stress. *Am J Clin Nutr*, 28:583, 1967.

28. Goetzl, E. J., Wasserman, S. I., and Ansten, K. F.: Enhancement of random migration and chemotactic response of human leukocytes by ascorbic acid. *J Clin Invest*, 53:813, 1974.

29. Wright, I. S. and MacLenathen, E.: Excretion of vitamin C in the sweat. *J Lab Clin Med*, 24:804, 1939.

30. Shields, J. B., Johnson, B. C., Hamilton, T. S., and Mitchell, H. H.: The excretion of ascorbic acid and dehydroascorbic acid in sweat and urine under different environmental conditions. *J Biol Chem*, 161:351, 1945.

31. Hindson, T. C.: Ascorbic acid status of Europeans resident in the tropics. *Br J Nutr*, 24:801, 1970.

32. Pelletier, O.: Vitamin C and cigarette smokers. *Ann NY Acad Sci*, 258:156, 1975.

33. Rowlands, J. R., Estefan, R. M., Gause, E. M., and Montalvo, D. A.: An electron spin resonance study of tobacco smoke condensates and their effects upon blood constituents. *Environ Res*, 2:47, 1968.

34. Young, D. L.: Relationships between cigarette smoking, oral contraceptives, and plasma vitamins A, E, and C, and plasma triglycerides and cholesterol. *Am J Clin Nutr*, 29:1216, 1976.

35. Nelson, M. N. and Farfar, J. O.: Associations between drugs admin-

istered during pregnancy and congenital abnormalities of the fetus. *Br Med J, 1*:523, 1971.

36. Goldsmith, G. A.: Human requirements for vitamin C and its use in clinical medicine. *Ann NY Acad Sci, 92*:230, 1961.

37. Scrimshaw, N. S.: *Nutrition and Stress in Diet and Bodily Constitution.* (G. E. W. Wolstenholme and M. O'Connor, Eds.) Ciba Foundation Study Group No. 17. Boston, Little, Brown and Co., 1964, p. 40.

38. Kyhos, E. D., Sevringhaus, E. L., and Hagedorn, D.: Large doses of ascorbic acid in treatment of vitamin C deficiencies. *Arch Intern Med, 75*:407, 1945.

39. Levenson, S. M., Green, R. W., Taylor, F. H. L., Robinson, P., Page, R. C., Johnson, R. E., and Lund, C. C.: Ascorbic acid, riboflavin, thiamine, and nicotinic acid in relation to severe injury, hemorrhage, and infection in the human. *Ann Surg, 124*:840, 1946.

40. Gerson, C. D.: Ascorbic acid deficiency in clinical disease, including regional euteritis. *Ann NY Acad Sci, 258*:483, 1975.

41. Maas, J. W., Gleser, G. C., and Gottschalk, L. A.: Schizophrenia, anxiety, and biochemical factors. *Arch Gen Psychiatry, 4*:109, 1961.

42. Milner, G.: Ascorbic acid in chronic psychiatric patients—a controlled trial. *Br J Psychiatry, 109*:294, 1963.

43. Bermond, P.: Clinical symptoms of malnutrition and plasma ascorbic acid levels. *Am J Clin Nutr, 29*:493, 1976.

44. Scarlett, J. A., Zeidler, A., Rockman, H., and Rubenstein, A.: Acute effect of ascorbic acid infusion on carbohydrate tolerance. *Am J Clin Nutr, 29*:1339, 1976.

45. Lamden, M. P. and Chrystowski, G. A.: Urinary oxalate excretion by man following ascorbic acid ingestion. *Proc Soc Exp Biol Med, 85*:190, 1954.

46. Briggs, M. N., Garcia-Webb, P., and Davies, P.: Urinary oxalate and vitamin C supplements. *Lancet, 2*:201, 1973.

47. Kean, W. F.: Vitamin C and the stone. *Lancet, 1*:364, 1974.

48. Stein, H. D., Hasan, A., and Fox, I. H.: Ascorbic acid-induced uricosuria. *Arch Intern Med, 84*:385, 1976.

VITAMIN D

Man has long known that fish liver contained healing substances. After the concept of accessory food factors—later called micronutrients—became established, the antirachitic property in fish liver oils was given the name "vitamin D" (although it was not ever believed to be an amine). The antirachitic effects of ultraviolet light in people added new aspects to the thinking about vitamin D. Early studies showed that the ultraviolet irradiation of some foods conferred antirachitic properties on them. When cholesterol in food was stated to become after irradiation the antirachitic property, the pronouncement was hailed as a great discovery. Soon, however, it became clear that it was not cholesterol but rather ergosterol, then believed to be an unimportant contaminant of cholesterol, that became vitamin D when irradiated. Vitamin D was then called viosterol. Later studies showed that there were a number of D-vitamins. One of the most powerful, formed by the irradiation of ergosterol, is now called vitamin D_2, and it bears the name "ergocalciferol." Another D-vitamin, equally potent, is vitamin D_3, formed by the action of ultraviolet in a cholesterol derivative, 7-dehydrocholesterol. This vitamin also bears the name "cholecalciferol." (There is no vitamin D_1.) However, recent studies have shown that vitamin D_2 and vitamin D_3 are physiologically inactive until they have been modified. They first accumulate in the liver, where an enzyme changes the D-vitamins to 25-hydroxyvitamin Ds. These then enter the bloodstream, and the serum level of 25-hydroxyvitamin D is measurable. (If an excess of vitamin D is taken by mouth, the 25-hydroxylation reaction ceases.) The serum compound, which is somewhat active, is further modified by hydroxylation in the kidney. If there is a need for calcium in the blood and tissues, the kidney adds a hydroxyl group at position 1, producing 1,25-dihydroxyvitamin D, the physiologically most active compound. If hypercalcemia develops, the kidney adds the hydroxyl group at position 24, producing 24-25-di-hydroxyvitamin D, which has little or no effect on calcium metabolism.

DeLuca, in whose laboratory many of the recent advances were made, has written a marvelously lucid account of how the vitamins D interact with parathyroid hormone in the regulation of calcium metabolism.[1]

One function of the active form of vitamin D is to secure the mineralization of bone, but this is not a direct effect. The vitamin does this by maintaining adequate amounts of calcium and inorganic phosphate at the calcification sites. The vitamin maintains appropriate calcium and phosphate concentrations by increasing intestinal absorption of both of them and, if necessary, by mobilizing both from calcified bone. (There is some evidence, not conclusive, that the vitamin increases the renal tubular reabsorption of calcium and phosphate.) The mobilization of calcium and phosphate from calcified bone depends both on vitamin D and on parathormone. It now appears that vitamin D not only secures the mineralization of osteod and cartilage but also helps maintain the serum calcium at normal levels. There is an intimate relation between vitamin D and parathormone actions. The formation of the 1,25-dihydroxyvitamin D depends on the presence of para-thormone, for it does not occur in parathyroidectomized animals until parathormone is given. In parathyroidectomized animals, the production of the 24,25 compound increases. The absorption of calcium from the intestine stimulated by 1,25-dihydroxyvitamin D is not affected by parathormone, but the action of the vitamin on bone requires the presence of parathormone. Thus, the role of parathormone in hypocalcemia is as follows: when the serum calcium level falls, the secretion of parathyroid hormone is stimulated. This hormone goes to the kidney where, among other things, it stimulates the formation of 1,25-dihydroxyvitamin D_3 and suppresses the formulation of 24,25-dihydroxyvitamin D. The 1,25 form goes to the intestine and stimulates absorption of calcium. When it goes to bone, it, together with parathyroid hormone, stimulates bone resorption. The place of hydroxylation at the 24 position in all this is now clear. Compounds hydroxylated in this position are rapidly metabolized and cleared from the body in the feces. These considerations explain not only dietary rickets and osteomalacia, but also the defects in calcium and phosphate metabolism produced by renal and hepatic disease. In addition, it must be remembered that the absorption of vitamin D from the intestine requires bile salts and pancreatic juices.

Except for fish-liver oils and eggs, vitamin D is not likely to be found in quantity in food. Hence, it is now put in milk in an amount of 400 units per quart. However, it deteriorates in the presence of mineral salts, and hence, in some countries a great deal more than 400 units may be added. (One milligram is equivalent to 40,000 units.)

The childhood type of vitamin D deficiency is hardly likely to be recognized by today's doctors in this country. In addition to the skeletal deformities that involve the extremities, the pelvis, the rib cage, and the head, there are other symptoms, such as generalized muscle weakness. The child with the disease is sick and fretful. Roentgenographic studies show demineralized bones. The serum 25-hydroxyvitamin D level, in the normal range in mild and early stages of the disease, falls to lower with increasing severity.[2] The blood calcium and inorganic phosphate levels may be low; if the former is sufficiently low, infantile tetany will develop. When vitamin D is given to children with rickets, it is important to give adequate amounts of calcium as well. If this is not done, the process of remineralization of bone may lower the serum calcium concentration to tetany levels.

A disorder of erythrocyte function also occurs in avitaminosis D. Over forty years ago Bakwin, Bodansky, and Turner[3] reported a decrease in certain phosphate compounds in the blood in rickets. A similar finding has recently been reported in adult vitamin D deficiency.[4] We now know that the compounds involved are ATP and 2,3-diphosphoglycertate. A lack of the former shortens the life span of red blood cells. A shortage of the latter impairs the ability of the red blood cells to unload oxygen in the tissues. In effect vitamin D deficiency causes tissue hypoxia in spite of normal oxygenation of the blood in the lungs.

The basic pathophysiologic process, failure of mineralization of osteoid and cartilage, may also occur in adult patients, and in them it causes osteomalacia.

Although the dietary form of vitamin D deficiency in American infants is uncommon, adults may develop it because of a poor diet or because of a malabsorption syndrome of some sort. The problem is complicated by the fact that some patients may have the abnormal serum calcium and phosphate levels and alkaline phosphatase activities characteristic of adult vitamin D deficiency and yet have no symptoms of it.[5] The biochemical disorder is cured by giving vitamin D. The occult vitamin D deficiency in this group was found to be more common in pregnant women. On the other hand, another study of women from India, this one conducted in England, produced different conclusions.[6] These authors also found low serum calcium levels in their pregnant subjects but ascribed it to hemodilution. Their finding of elevated serum alkaline phosphatase levels they declared to be the result of over-production of this enzyme by the placenta. The figures for serum 25-hydroxyvitamin D level did not change during pregnancy, and the authors concluded that their patients did not have vitamin D deficiency. This reliance on a single laboratory finding, one that measures not the most active compound (1,25-dihydroxyvitamin D) but only an intermediate, is somewhat disconcerting. Other results of the study showed values lower in Asians than Caucasians, and especially low values in Asian vegetarians.[6] The significance of these findings cannot be stated. A study made in another Asian group, Bedouins, had significantly lower serum 25-hydroxyvitamin D levels than did Caucasians.[7] There again, pregnant women had lower levels than the non-pregnant, but never within what is believed to be the deficiency range.

On the other hand, severe protracted infections may produce rickets despite what appears to be an adequate intake.[8] The utilization is decreased or the requirement increased owing to factors not yet clarified. The absorption of the vitamin has been measured and found low in malabsorption syndromes.[9] The liver is clearly important in the transformation of vitamin D to 25-hydroxyvitamin D. Patients with cirrhosis and with celiac disease have low serum values of 25-hydroxyvitamin D. (Alcoholics without recognizable liver disease generally do not.) After an intravenous dose of vitamin D, the level rises in normal subjects and celiac patients, but not in patients with cirrhosis.[10] Magnesium deficiency, such as occurs in certain gastrointestinal diseases and in some alcoholic patients, may cause hypocalcemia that does not respond to vitamin D but does disappear with magnesium depletion.[11]

It is now the custom, when someone makes a discovery, for a great number of authors to publish papers on the same subject. The discovery that anticonvulsant drugs cause rickets and osteomalacia quickly led to the development of a large literature on the subject. Four papers published in 1975 and 1976[12, 13, 14, 15] give us the latest information. Either diphenylhydantoin or phenobarbital, or both taken together, has been found to cause small changes in serum calcium, serum inorganic phosphate, serum 25-hydroxyvitamin D concentration and in calcified bone mass as measured. However, the serum alkaline phosphatase activity is markedly increased. The measured calcified bone mass did not seem to correlate well with the roentgenographic appearance of rickets or osteomalacia. The literature records great disagreement about the dose of vitamin D necessary to cure the disorder—the recommended doses ranging from 1,000 units per day to several times that. It is possible that where the doses in this range were ineffective, either complicating factors were present or else the dietary calcium was not adequately increased.

Toxic effects occur with large doses of vitamin D. Time is a factor in this process, as is the age of the subject. Giving as little as 20,000 units a day for several months may kill a child, but adults tolerate doses several times as large. Symptoms of toxicity are anorexia, polyuria, weight loss, and signs of renal disease. Later, headache, vomiting, lassitude, and signs of uremia develop. Metastatic calcification may be widespread, but the involvement of the arteries of parenchymal organs, especially the kidneys, is most damaging. Long after the toxic doses are discontinued, evidence of renal impairment may exist. The metastatic calcification may occur without hypercalcemia. One author adduced evidence that prolonged ingestion of vitamin D causes myocardial infarction.[16] The data suggested that a daily intake of 30 micrograms or more might be critical.

RECOMMENDATIONS

There are no recommended daily amounts for vitamin D. Children taking anticonvulsant drugs should probably be given 1,000 units daily, with adults taking twice as much. In other conditions the requirement is variable, and hence, each patient given the vitamin in large doses must be closely supervised.

REFERENCES

1. DeLuca, H. F.: Recent advances in our understanding of the vitamin D endocrine system. *J Lab Clin Med, 87*:7, 1975.
2. Armand, S. B., Stickler, G. B., and Haworth, J. C.: Serum 25-hydroxyvitamin D in infantile rickets. *Pediatrics, 57*:221, 1976.
3. Bakwin, H., Bodansky, O., and Turner, R.: Phosphorus components in the blood of normal and rachitic infants. *Proc Soc Exp Biol Med, 36*:365, 1937.
4. Love, E. W. and Morgan, D. B.: The effect of vitamin D on phosphates in human red blood cells and in tissues of the chick. *Comp Biochem Physiol, 44B*:557, 1973.
5. Rab, S. M. and Baseer, A.: Occult osteomalacia amongst healthy and pregnant women in Pakistan. *Lancet, 2*:1211, 1976.
6. Dent, C. E. and Gupta, M. M.: Plasma 25-hydroxyvitamin-D levels during pregnancy in Caucasians and in vegetarian and non-vegetarian Asians. *Lancet, 2*:1057, 1975.
7. Shany, S., Hirsh, J., and Berlyne, G. M.: 25-hydroxycholecalciferol levels in Bedouins in the Niger. *Am J Clin Nutr, 29*:1104, 1976.
8. Park, E. A.: The influence of severe illness on rickets. *Arch Dis Child, 29*:369, 1954.
9. Thompson, G. W., Lewis, B., and Booth, C. C.: Asborption of vitamin D_3^{-3H} in control subjects and patients with intestinal malabsorption. *J Clin Invest, 45*:94, 1966.
10. Hepner, G. W., Roginsky, M., and Moo, H. F.: Abnormal vitamin D metabolism in patients with cirrhosis. *Digest Dis, 21*:527, 1976.
11. Medalle, R., Waterhouse, C., and Hahn, T. J.: Vitamin D resistance in magnesium deficiency. *Am J Clin Nutr, 29*:834, 1976.
12. Hahn, T. J., Hendon, B. A., Scharp, C. R., Boisseau, V. C., and Haddad, J. C.: Serum 25-hydroxycalciferol levels and bone mass in children on chronic anticonvulsant therapy. *New Engl J Med, 292*:550, 1975.
13. Christiansen, C., Rodbro, P., Munck, O., and Munck, O.: Actions of vitamins D_2 and D_3 and 25-OHD$_3$ in anticonvulsant osteomalacia. *Br Med J, 1*:363, 1975.
14. Peterson, P., Gray, P., and Tolman, K. G.: Calcium balance in drug-

induced osteomalacia: Response to vitamin D. *Clin Pharmacol Ther, 19*:63, 1976.

15. Mosekilde, L. and Melsen, F.: Anticonvulsant osteomalacia determined by quantitative analysis of bone changes. *Acta Med Scand, 199*:349, 1976.

16. Linden, V.: Vitamin D and myocardial infarction. *Br Med J, 2*:647, 1974.

TOCOPHEROL – VITAMIN E

T HE BIOLOGICAL ROLE of vitamin E remains obscure despite a vast amount of biochemical research, both at tissue and subcellular levels. There is no doubt that vitamin E deficiency causes in some species sterility in males, absorption of the fetus in females, severe muscular dystrophy both peripheral and cardiac, liver necrosis, anemia, neurological disorders, and a number of less well-defined syndromes. Although some authors have maintained that vitamin E acts only as an antioxidant, it now seems clear that in a deficiency of the vitamin ordinary antioxidants cannot replace it entirely. The situation with respect to human deficiency is most obscure.

Vitamin E actually consists of a considerable number of tocopherols and related substances that have vitamin E activity.[1] These compounds are widely distributed in nature, but man obtains them chiefly from vegetable fats. Alpha-tocopherol is a highly potent vitamin E substance, but today Americans obtain increasing amounts of the vitamin in the much less potent form of gamma-tocopherol[2] because of the loss of alpha-tocopherol in food processing. The complex relations between vitamin E and lipid metabolism in man were noted many years ago.[3] The requirement for vitamin E is now recognized to be related to the tissue content of polyunsaturated lipid, and the latter is changed (depending on the tissue) rapidly or slowly.[4] A masterly discussion of the problems involved in establishing criteria for vitamin E intake was recently published by Horwitt.[5] A well-fed adult in this country apparently carries approximately a four-year supply of the vitamin in his liver and adipose tissues. A well-fed person on a diet that contains small amounts of polyunsaturated fatty acids would probably do well on 15 I.U. per day of dietary alpha-tocopherol whereas a person taking a large amount of polyunsaturated fatty acid would do poorly on two or three times that dose. The situation is complicated by the fact that people or animals on very low intakes of unsaturated fatty acids will synthesize them. Horwitt's calculations[5] led him to conclude that between 10 and 30 mg of alpha-tocopherol covered the adult requirements. However, different tocopherols have different potencies, some of them being very weak.[6] The blood level at birth is low, but quickly rises to adult levels.[7]

Vitamin E is believed to protect vitamins A and C, carotene, and selenium against oxidation in the gut, but little is known about this action.

As we would expect, rapidly growing organisms need larger amounts of vitamin E than do adults. The observations of Horwitt et al.[8] on the anemia of vitamin E deficiency naturally led to the search for this anemia in infants. It now seems established that the anemia of premature infants is largely due to this deficiency.[9] The anemia developed within two weeks after the diet was changed from human to cow's milk. In this study the standard method of evaluating the effect of vitamin E deficiency was used; namely, to measure the susceptibility of the red blood cells to hemolysis by peroxide. This hemolysis increased when the blood vitamin E level was below 0.6 mg per 100 ml. The role of artificial diets in this anemia was discussed in a recent report[10] that showed that artificial formulae were so rich in unsaturated fatty acids as to become inadequate with respect to vitamin E content. A question naturally arises about another syndrome of premature infants, i.e. retrolental fibroplasia. A recent study[11] indicates that vitamin E supplementation of the diet reduces the severity and long-term morbidity of this disease. It is evident that the vitamin E is more important in infants given the excessive oxygen therapy formerly used than in those not given it.

The possibility that vitamin E might prevent the effects of our pollution by ozone has been studied in animals but not in man.

In adult persons the situation is far less clear. Definite vitamin E deficiency was formerly seen only in some adult patients with malabsorption syndromes. Today, with large numbers of persons taking excessive amounts of polyunsaturated acids for super-stitious reasons, the situation is different. Earlier studies in man showed that anemia occurred in vitamin E deficiency and that it was associated with abnormal susceptibility to hemolysis by hydrogen peroxide. However, this sensitive test is rarely performed except in a few research groups. Nor are serum levels, probably less reliable, often measured. The true incidence of vitamin E deficiency in adult man is not known.

A few decades ago vitamin E began to be recommended for the treatment or prevention of atherosclerosis, phlebitis, and other vascular disorders. This recommendation apparently was extrapolated from the observation that vitamin E benefited the symptoms of atherosclerosis of the legs. As a matter of fact, vitamin E does ameliorate intermittent claudication. This conclusion is based not only on the clinical observations of a number of competent clinicians but also on biopsy studies[12] and blood-flow measurements of the muscles of patients with ischemia of the leg muscles. Biopsy studies showed that patients with this disorder have low vitamin E concentrations in the involved muscles and exhibit diminished blood flows in them. Giving vitamin E in a dose of 300 mg (approximately 450 units) a day caused improved blood flows and an increase in the vitamin E level in the muscles. In these studies the vitamin E was given for longer periods than in some earlier reports. On the other hand, the results of relatively short-term observations in coronary atherosclerosis do not support the view that vitamin E is beneficial in treating the symptoms of coronary atherosclerosis.[13-15] Nevertheless, when patients who had been taking vitamin E for a long time were given an undistinguishable placebo instead, more than half became worse.[15] The situation with respect to coronary atherosclerosis is now changed, however. Now that many patients with this disease are taking large amounts of polyunsaturated fatty acids for superstitious reasons, a large intake of vitamin E is mandatory.

Another idea that comes to the fore from time to time is that because vitamin E deficiency causes muscular dystrophy in many animals, taking an excess should improve muscle function in man. Giving 900 units a day for six months had no such effect.[16]

Estrogen is known to affect serum lipid levels, and hence, studies have been made on vitamin E concentrations in patients taking oral contraceptives.[17, 18] Estrogen causes no change or a small rise in the serum vitamin E level.

The possibility that vitamin E may be toxic when taken in large amounts must be considered. There are few data bearing on this subject. In one study a total of 296,000 mg of alpha-tocopherol was given to a man over a three-month period with no detectable clinical evidences of toxicity.[19] However, more recent authors have reported the development of a poorly defined feeling of fatigue in their subjects who took much less.

Another effect, which might be considered either good or bad depending on one's bias, is prolongation of the clotting time.[6] This is a consequence of the formation of hydroquinones by oxidation of the vitamin E. These oxides inhibit the action of vitamin K.

RECOMMENDATIONS

Although milling removes much of the vitamin E from grains and cereals consumed in this country, there is nothing to indicate the occurrence of a deficiency in man except for infants on formulas, patients with malabsorption syndromes, and persons who take large amounts of polyunsaturated fatty acids.

For adults in the above categories, doses of 600 units per day (or more) appear to be reasonable.

REFERENCES

1. Hoffmann-Ostenhof, O.: Problems in the stereochemical designation of tocopherols and related compounds. *Am J Clin Nutr, 27*:1105, 1974.
2. Bieri, J. G. and Evarts, R. P.: Gamma tocopherol: Metabolism, biological activity, and significance in human vitamin E nutrition. *Am J Clin Nutr, 27*:980, 1974.
3. Horwitt, M. K.: Vitamins and lipid metabolism in man. *Am J Clin Nutr, 8*:451, 1960.
4. Witting, L. A.: Vitamin E—Polyunsaturated lipid relationship in diet and tissues. *Am J Clin Nutr, 27*:952, 1974.
5. Horwitt, M. K.: Studies of human requirements for vitamin E. *Am J Clin Nutr, 27*:1182, 1974.
6. Horwitt, M. K.: Vitamin E: a reexamination. *Am J Clin Nutr, 29*:569, 1976.
7. Vobecky, J. S., Vobecky, J., Shapcott, D., and Blanchard, R.: Vitamin E and C levels in infants during the first year of life. *Am J Clin Nutr, 29*:766, 1976.
8. Horwitt, M. R., Harvey, C. C., Duncan, G. D., and Harvey, W. C.: Effects of limited tocopherol intake in man with relationship to

erythrocyte hemolysis and lipid oxidations. *Am J Clin Nutr, 8*:451, 1960.

9. Lo, S. S., Frank, D., and Hitzig, W. H.: Vitamin E and hemolytic anaemia in premature infants. *Arch Dis Child, 48*:360, 1973.

10. Davis, K. C.: Vitamin E: adequacy of infant diets. *Am J Clin Nutr, 25*:953, 1972.

11. Johnson, L., Schaffer, D., and Boggs, T. R., Jr.: The premature infant, vitamin E deficiency and retrolental fibroplasia. *Am J Clin Nutr, 27*:1158, 1974.

12. Haeger, K.: Long-time treatment of intermittent claudication with vitamin E. *Am J Clin Nutr, 27*:1179, 1974.

13. Olson, R. E.: Vitamin E and its relation to heart disease. *Circulation, 48*:179, 1973.

14. Hodges, R. E.: Are there any indications for vitamin E in the treatment of cardiovascular diseases? *Drug Therapy, 3*:101, 1973.

15. Anderson, T. W., and Reid, D. B. W.: A double-blind trial of vitamin E in angina pectoris. *Am J Clin Nutr, 27*:1174, 1974.

16. Lawrence, J. D., Bower, R. C., Riehl, W. P., and Smith, J. L.: Effects of a tocopherol acetate on the swimming endurance of trained swimmers. *Am J Clin Nutr, 28*:205, 1975.

17. Young, D. L. and Chan, P. L.: Effects of a progestogen and a sequential type of oral contraceptive on plasma vitamin A, vitamin E, cholesterol, and triglycerides. *Am J Clin Nutr, 28*:686, 1975.

18. Young, D. L.: Relationships between cigarette smoking, oral contraceptives, and plasma vitamins A, E, C, and plasma triglycerides and cholesterol. *Am J Clin Nutr, 29*:1216, 1976.

19. Hilman, R. W.: Tocopherol excess in man. Creatinuria associated with prolonged ingestion. *Am J Clin Nutr, 5*:597, 1957.

VITAMIN K

THE SITUATION WITH respect to vitamin K is anomalous in that it is probably the least understood of the vitamins biochemically and yet by far the one most often studied in clinical practice. A scholarly series of papers in *The Fat-Soluble Vitamins*, edited by DeLuca and Suttie, presents the results of many biochemical studies, but tells us little that explains the vitamin's role in clinical medicine.[1]

What is known is that the vitamin is fat-soluble, that bile must be present in the intestine for the vitamin to be absorbed, that once absorbed it is carried to the liver, and that in the liver it stimulates in some unknown way the synthesis of prothrombin (factor II), proconvertin (factor VII), Christmas factor (factor IX) and Stuart factor (factor X). These are all blood-clotting factors, and some authorities hold that some or all of them are merely variants of one plasma protein.

The relation of prothrombin to liver function is evident. Bile is needed for the absorption of vitamin K, and the vitamin K makes the clotting factors in the liver. Where the liver is abnormal in function, administered vitamin K is powerless to stimulate it to make the clotting factors. These mechanisms come into play in bile-duct obstruction and in parenchymatous liver disease. Vitamin K, by injection, is highly effective in the former and poorly effective, or ineffective, in the latter. It is appropriate that the substance be called vitamin K for *Koagulation*.

The vitamin exists in several forms, all with a 1,4 naphthoquinone nucleus but with different side chains. The active form in animals has a methyl and a geranylgeranyl side chain and is called vitamin K_2. The vitamin is found in various forms in leafy plants, walnuts, henna, plumbago, and in decaying fish. A derivative, menadione, also called vitamin K_3, is used in medicine, often as a water-soluble derivative.

157

In addition to diseases of the liver and bile ducts, vitamin K deficiency may also occur in malabsorption syndromes and chronic diarrheal diseases. It also appears to be the cause of neonatal hemorrhage.

Its only clinical manifestations are hemorrhagic.

In clinical practice, aside from the conditions listed, it occurs commonly, produced by design, in a controlled degree in patients given warfarin in the treatment of phlebitis or myocardial infarction. The structure of warfarin indicates that it counteracts vitamin K by competition.

RECOMMENDATIONS

To control the hemorrhagic disorder of liver or biliary disease rapidly, the vitamin is given by injection. When it is necessary to give it for prolonged periods, the dose is 2 mg per day, given together with bile salts.

REFERENCES

1. DeLuca, H. F. and Suttie, J. W.: *The Fat-Soluble Vitamins.* Madison, University of Wisconsin Press, 1969.

PART V

MISCELLANEOUS TOPICS

TOXIC SUBSTANCES TAKEN IN
OR WITH FOOD

T HE VAST NUMBER of toxic substances that may be taken in or with food fall into several categories.

1. Poisonous substances that occur normally in plants and animals, exemplified by the poisons found in some mushrooms and in a number of exotic fishes. They are not likely to be eaten by people who know what they are about. They will not be discussed here.

2. Substances formed by molds and bacteria in food after harvesting, presale processing, or cooking. These range from the cancer-producing afflatoxins of moldy peanuts or grain to the staphlococcal toxins of certain badly refrigerated foods. These, too, will not be discussed here because food poisoning is not a nutritional problem.

3. Food additives—colorants, preservatives, and antioxidants —that remain in the food eaten by the consumer. They will not be discussed here. The reader will find fuller information elsewhere.[1]

4. Female hormones given to cattle and formerly implanted in capons to make them fatter. Although these are carcinogenic when taken in large amounts, it is not likely that they have this, or any other, deleterious effect in man. Nevertheless, diethylstilbesterol, the one most commonly used, is atherogenic, and one wonders whether it contributes to the high incidence of atherosclerosis in affluent countries. Moreover, since it is feminizing, one also wonders what effect it is having in a generation of young men brought up on hamburger patties and fried chicken.

5. Organic insecticides and pesticides which remain in the food eaten by the consumer.

Chlorophenothane (DDT) is the oldest of the modern insecticides and, hence, the most studied. The chemical is now widely distributed in mammalian and avian species and accumulates particularly in fat. Many studies have been made in which DDT has been fed to experimental animals; in some of these animals neoplasms developed. The significance of these findings for human health cannot be stated because malignant tumors will develop in one mammalian species or another if almost any substance is given in sufficiently large amounts. Also, there is clear evidence that the reproductive functions of birds living in nature are affected adversely after the ingestion of DDT in relatively small amounts, but this has not been shown to occur in man.

As regards man, there is no doubt that the chemical is accumulating in body fat, but no adverse effects have yet been demonstrated. The most disquieting finding in this connection is the discovery that human milk contains DDT.[2, 3] Data obtained in a number of cities and rural areas in this country show that the milk of nursing human mothers contains amounts many times greater than the concentration permitted in cow's milk.[2, 3] Milk obtained at the beginning of each nursing contains much more DDT than milk obtained at the end. In addition, the older the mother and the more children she has nursed, the lower the DDT level in her milk.[2] No environmental factors have been proved responsible for the high DDT levels in human milk. However, in one study the levels were lower in women who hired exterminators than in women who used household insecticides.[2] A more definite factor was the eating of margarine instead of butter. The margarine eaters produced milk with levels of DDT twice that of the butter eaters. (Margarine is made from corn oil, and DDT is extensively used to protect the corn corp.) In the rural subjects the nearby dusting of crops was a factor.[3]

There is no evidence to indicate that drinking DDT-contaminated mothers' milk has done any children any harm. Perhaps it is too early to recognize possible far-reaching effects.

6. Chemicals normally present in food which may be dangerous in certain amounts under certain circumstances. These include oxalates (discussed elsewhere), nitrates, and phosphates.

Nitrates and nitrites have received alarming attention at intervals during the past three or four decades. On the average, an American eats about 300 gm of vegetables per day, containing about 85 mg of nitrate. More than half of this amount is supplied by 30 gm of leafy vegetables. Part of the ingested nitrate is put out in the saliva, where some of it is changed to nitrite—about 9 or 10 mg of this substance. This is approximately four times as much as that obtained from an average intake of cured meats in one day. Around the middle of the present century, nitrates and their oxidation products, the nitrites, were much discussed as the cause of methemoglobinemia in infants, who are particularly susceptible. This condition was recognized by the greyish cyanosis, dyspnea, and tachycardia caused by the action of the chemicals on the blood hemoglobin. In most cases the nitrate was in well water contaminated by surface runoff containing the chemical. In some cases, however, the cause was believed to be spinach fed the infants.[4]

A great furor was stirred up in this country recently because nitrates are added to meats during curing. Oxidation of nitrate to nitrite, and some subsequent chemical reactions in the intestinal tract, may lead to the formation of nitrosamines, which are known to be carcinogenic. Cured meats are permitted to contain only 200 parts per million of nitrate, which is supposed to lower the risk. The importance of this fact is somewhat diminished by the well-known data on nitrates in vegetables, many of which contain this much or even very much more. The vegetables with the highest amounts are beets, squash, parsley, turnips, radishes, celery, cabbage, lettuce, spinach, stringbeans, and eggplant.[4] In some parts of the world, vegetables contain dangerous amounts of nitrite because of having been grown on soils deficient in molybdenum. During storage much of this nitrate in vegetables turns to nitrite. The change to nitrite is prevented by vitamin C,[5, 6, 7] and this is found in all plants. However, the vitamin may be destroyed by oxidation during storage or cooking. The taking of supplementary vitamin C prevents nitrite formation.

The cancerophobia that now prevails in this country has undoubtedly led to an exaggeration of the dangers of cured meats, such as bacon. The customary taking of citrus fruit juice with this expensive breakfast food should abolish any hazards associated with eating it. The high nitrate content of some vegetables deserves more consideration, and the taking of supplemental vitamin C is a reasonable solution.

Phosphates have received little attention as sources of possible harm. Nevertheless, the taking of excessive amounts of phosphate in the diet, i.e. enough to raise the intake of phosphate well above the optimal intake equal to that of the intake of calcium, distorts calcium metabolism. Intakes of phosphate that approach or exceed double the normal, i.e. that reach or exceed 2.0 grams per day, clearly stimulate the parathyroid glands.[8] It is probable that lesser amounts do so also. This parathyroid hyperfunction is held by some to be responsible in part for the loss of bone substance that occurs with aging. Certain processed foods are responsible for the changes reported. Excessive intakes of phosphate occur when processed cheese is substituted for natural cheese, processed meats for natural meats, fabricated potato chips for natural potato chips, refrigerator quick rolls for yeast bread and rolls, refrigerator fruit turnovers for fruit pies, and certain carbonated beverages for citric-acid containing beverages.

7. Metals taken inadvertently with food, or deliberately as part of a dietary regimen. These are highly important as causes of disease. Three metals will be considered here: aluminum, cadmium, and lead. If they have any nutritional function, it is unknown, and beyond certain limits of intake, they are toxic.

Aluminum. A few years ago the findings of increased amounts of aluminum in the brain lesions of Alzheimer's disease[9, 10] stimulated much interest. This occurred at a time when our conception of Alzheimer's disease had begun to change. It was formerly considered an uncommon disorder and called "presenile psychosis," but the discovery in recent years that the lesions of the common senile psychosis were the same but less severe than in Alzheimer's disease has led many physicians to conclude that the two were really the same disease.

There is no way of knowing today whether the abnormal accumulation of aluminum found in the brain is cause or effect. A new interest in the subject developed after the reports of a correlation between brain aluminum content and the development of dementia in patients with total renal failure who were being kept alive by dialysis. It is customary to give such patients large amounts of aluminum hydroxide in order to limit the absorption of phosphate from the gut. This literature has recently been reviewed by Alfrey et al.[11]

A question naturally arises whether the ingestion of large amounts of aluminum gels as part of an anti-ulcer regimen over a period of many years can also cause serious aluminum retention. It does not.[12]

Cadmium. This metal is a highly dangerous industrial contaminant. It is being considered here because formerly the metal was regularly used in ice-cube trays, and significant amounts of the metal may have been ingested unknowingly. One of the most interesting manifestations of subclinical cadmium intoxication is the development of atherosclerosis.[13] This occurs in association with a *lowering* of the serum cholesterol level. It is interesting to conjecture whether the increasing incidence of coronary artery disease in the recent past, an epidemic that has mysteriously begun to abate, may have been a late result of the ingestion years ago of the cadmium in refrigerator ice trays, the recent decrease in the incidence of atherosclerosis being due to a change in the materials used.

One of the effects of cadmium intoxication, still a danger in industry, is the development of anemia. This seems to be aggravated by large amounts of vitamin B_6,[14] and hence, this vitamin should be given with great caution to persons exposed to possible industrial toxicity of cadmium.

Lead. Lead poisoning is a familiar disorder. It is commonly caused by pica in malnourished children and is not usually considered a nutritional disorder. Nevertheless, a considerable amount of lead may enter the body in nutriment. Lead in food ordinarily represents the major source of the metal that enters the body.[15, 16] Most of the lead enters food from the soil, but surface contamination of fruits and vegetables sold from open stands near busy highways also occurs. This may make a significant contribution to the lead ingested.

More dangerous in the development of lead toxicity is absorption of the metal into acid foods served in cheap pottery with lead-containing glazes. This hazard was described in detail 250 years ago[17] and is customarily ignored until another epidemic calls it to mind, as occurred a few years ago. The recent interest in folk craft led to the epidemic of a few years ago in this country.

The old practice of sweetening cider with sugar of lead

(lead acetate) is forbidden in civilized countries but probably still occurs in out-of-the-way places.

8. Food-packaging materials.

Phthalates. Phthalate esters are used to render plastics pliable. Without so-called *plasticizers,* plastics used as containers, e.g. vinyl plastics, would be so brittle as to be unusable for most purposes. Approximately 18 million pounds of vinyl plastics made flexible with phthalates are used as food wrappers or containers. However, nonphthalate-containing plastics, e.g. polyethylene, polypropylene, and styrene plastics, are also widely used. Phthalates may be ingested with food which has absorbed it from its covering, or from some such food as fish that has taken in the plastic from its environment.

There is no evidence that, in the amounts that could possibly be taken in, toxic effects from phthalate ingestion can occur.[18]

REFERENCES

1. *The Use of Chemicals in Food Production, Processing, Storage, and Distribution.* A report of the Subcommittee on Food Technology of the Food and Nutrition Board. NAS-NRC, Washington, D.C., 34 pp.
2. Wilson, D. J., Locker, D. J., Ritzen, C. A., Watson, J. T., and Schaffner, W.: DDT concentrations in human milk. *Am J Dis Child, 125*:814, 1973.
3. Woodward, B. T., Ferguson, B. B., and David, P.: DDT levels in milk of rural indigent blacks. *Am J Dis Child, 30*:400, 1976.
4. Lee, D. H. K.: Nitrates, nitrites, and methemoglobinemia. *Environ Res, 3*:484, 1970.
5. Kamm, J. J., Dashman, T., Conney, A. H., and Burns, J. J.: Effect of ascorbic acid on amine-nitrite toxicity. *Ann NY Acad Sci, 258*:169, 1975.
6. Mirvish, S. S.: Blocking the formation of N-nitroso compounds with ascorbic acid *in vitro* and *in vivo. Ann NY Acad Sci, 258*:169, 1975.
7. Raineri, R. and Weisburger, J. H.: Reduction of gastric carcinogens with ascorbic acid. *Ann NY Acad Sci, 258*:181, 1975.
8. Bell, R. R., Draper, H. H., Tzeng, D. Y. M., Shin, H. K., and Schmidt, C. R.: Physiological responses of human adults to foods containing phosphate additives. *J Nutr, 107*:42, 1977.
9. Crapper, D. R., Krishnan, S. S., and Dalton, A. J.: Brain aluminum distribution in Alzheimer's disease and experimental neurofibrillary

degeneration. *Science, 180*:511, 1973.

10. Crapper, D. R., Krishnan, S. S., and Quittkatt, S.: Aluminum, neurofibrillary degeneration and Alzheimer's disease. *Brain, 99*:67, 1976.
11. Alfrey, A. C., Le Gendre, G. R., and Kaehny, W. D.: The dialysis encephalopathy syndrome. Possible aluminum intoxication. *N Engl J Med, 294*:184, 1976.
12. Cam, J. M., Luck, V. A., Eastwood, J. B., and deWardener, H. E.: The effect of aluminum hydroxide orally on calcium, phosphorus and aluminum metabolism in normal subjects. *Clin Sci Mol Med, 51*:407, 1976.
13. Schroeder, H. A. and Balassa, J. J.: Influence of chromium, cadmium, and lead on the rat, aortic lipids and circulating cholesterol. *Am J Physiol, 209*:433, 1965.
14. Stowe, H. D., Goyen, R. A., Medley, P., and Cates, M.: Influence of dietary pyridoxine on cadmium toxicity in rats. *Arch Environ Health, 28*:209, 1974.
15. Waldron, H. A.: Subclinical lead poisoning: a preventable disease. *Preventive Medicine, 4*:135, 1975.
16. Ter Haar, G., Dedolph, R. R., Holtzman, R. B., and Lucas, H. F., Jr.: The lead uptake by perennial ryegrass and radishes from air, water and soil. *Environ Res, 2*:267, 1969.
17. Baker, G.: An examination of several means, by which the poison of Lead may be supposed frequently to gain admittance into the human body, unobserved, and unsuspected. In *Medical Transactions,* London, College of Physicians, *1*:257, 1768.
18. Phthalates in food. A scientific status summary by the Institute of Food Technologists' Expert Panel on Food Safety and Nutrition and The Committee on Public Information. *Nutr Rev, 32*:126, 1974.

DIETARY FIBER (ROUGHAGE)

For MANY DECADES patients with chronic constipation have been told to eat more roughage, including, if necessary, the roughage removed from food in processing, i.e. bran. In the past, patients with a wide variety of gastrointestinal disorders, e.g. gastritis, peptic ulcer, irritable colon, ileitis, colitis, diverticulosis, were ordered to abjure roughage even though the food containing it might have been turned to mush by cooking. Some such patients were told to eat no vegetables except as purees. The validity of this advice has recently been questioned.

The subject of dietary fiber has recently received much attention, and the result has been an excess of comment combined with a deficiency of data. Good review articles are available.[1, 2]

A distinction must be made between dietary fiber—any vegetable material that resists digestion in the human intestinal tract—and so-called *crude fiber*. The latter is a chemists' concept and refers to what is left after treatment with boiling sulphuric acid, strong alkali, water, alcohol, and ether. This obviously has little to do with human nutrition. A classification of plant fibers as they apply to nutrition was recently put forward by Spiller et al.[3] Its use should help to minimize the confusion that now exists in this field.

Dietary fiber consists of celluloses, water-soluble hemicelluloses, lignin, and probably other substances. When present in cooked food, fiber may or may not look fibrous and is not necessarily even tough. The American diet contains 8 or 10 grams per day; the British diet, a little more than half that. In the last century and a half, there has been a considerable decrease in fiber intake derived from grains and, on the whole, some increase in fiber derived from fruits and vegetables. Cummings' report[1] discusses the chemistry and physiology of dietary fiber in detail.

Recent interest in dietary fiber rose out of a negative correlation between its intake and diverticular disease of the colon.[4, 5] The slowed transit time and increased intraluminal pressure associated with the low residue diet are believed to lead to diverticulosis. Other authors have stressed the relationship between the irritable colon syndrome and diverticulosis.[6, 7] On the other hand, in some studies no correlation between roughage and colon disease has been found.[8] Nevertheless, the evidence as regards diverticulosis is convincing.

Other studies have related a low residue diet not only to colonic disease but to hemorrhoids, gallstones, hiatal hernias, abdominal hernias, and varicose veins.[9] The effect of one fiber, bran, in the diet is reported to cause the bile to be less saturated with cholesterol than before.[10] This change, which retards gallstone formation, appears to be due to an increased synthesis of chenodeoxycholate.[10] These observations deserve repeated replication as well as extension to other types of fiber. It has been known for years that one form of fiber, pectin, in the diet lowers serum cholesterol level somewhat. This observation was recently recorded again.[11] There is no reason to accept the notion, uttered by the uncritical, that this will have any effect on coronary artery disease. The evidence concerning these other diseases, and also colonic cancer, is not convincing.[1, 2, 12]

An obvious way to add fiber to the diet is to feed wheat bran. However, there is a great deal of difference in the effects of bran when taken as the commercially available material, as bran seived from whole wheat flour, and as whole wheat bread itself.[13-16] With the coarser preparations, fecal fat excretion increases, and calcium with it. The serum iron and folate levels may fall. In addition, eating wheat bran causes decreased absorption of calcium, magnesium, zinc, and phosphorus.[17] It also causes trifling decreases in serum lipid levels.[14]

Although the low residue diet formerly used to treat the irritable colon syndrome, colonic diverticulosis, and gallbladder disease may have been ill advised, there is no reason to go to the opposite extreme and prescribe the visibly coarsest forms of roughage.

RECOMMENDATIONS

Fruits and vegetables, cooked or raw, should be included in the diet in considerable amounts. The addition of bran as such, or the use of the coarsest breads in the diet, is ill advised.

REFERENCES

1. Cummings, J. H.: Progress report. Dietary fiber. *Gut, 14*:69, 1973.
2. Mendeloff, A. I.: Dietary fiber. *Nutr Rev, 33*:321, 1975.
3. Spiller, G. A., Fassett-Cornelius, G., and Briggs, G. M.: A new term for plant fibres in nutrition. *Am J Clin Nutr, 29*:934, 1976.
4. Painter, N. S. and Burkitt, D. P.: Diverticular disease of the colon: A deficiency disease of Western civilization. *Br Med J, 1*:450, 1971.
5. Segal, I., Solomon, A., and Hunt, J. A.: Emergence of diverticular disease in the urban South African black. *Gastroenterology, 73*:215, 1977.
6. Berman, P. M. and Kirsner, J. B.: Diverticular disease of the colon—the possible role of "roughage" in both food and life. *Am J Dig Dis, 18*:506, 1973.
7. Reilly, R. W. and Kirsner, J. B.: Fiber deficiency and colonic disorders. *Am J Clin Nutr, 28*:293, 1975.
8. Dorfman, S. H., Ali, M., and Floch, M. H.: Low fiber content of Connecticut diets. *Am J Clin Nutr, 29*:87, 1976.
9. Brodribb, J. M. and Humphreys, D. M.: Diverticular disease: Three studies. Part 1. Relation to other diseases and fiber intake. *Br Med J, 1*:424, 1976.
10. Pomare, E. W., Heaton, K. W., Low-beer, T. S., and Espiner, H. J.: The effect of wheat bran upon bile salt metabolism and upon the lipid composition of bile in gallstone patients. *Dig Dis, 21*:521, 1976.
11. Durrington, P. N., Manning, A. P., Bolton, C. N., and Hartog, M.: Effect of pectin on serum lipids and lipoproteins, whole-gut transit time, and stool weight. *Lancet, 2*:394, 1976.
12. Alcantara, E. N. and Speckmann, E. W.: Diet, nutrition, and cancer. *Am J Clin Nutr, 29*:1035, 1976.
13. Kirwan, W. O., Smith, A. W., McConnell, A. A., Mitchell, W. D., and Eastwood, J. B.: Action of different bran preparations on colonic function. *Br Med J, 1*:187, 1974.
14. Jenkins, D. J. A., Hill, M. S., and Cummings, J. H.: Effect of wheat fiber on blood lipids, fecal steroid excretion, and serum iron. *Am J Clin Nutr, 28*:1408, 1975.
15. Brodribb, J. M. and Humphreys, D. M.: Diverticular disease: Three

studies. Part III. Metabolic effects of bran in patients with diverticular disease. *Br Med J, 1*:428, 1976.

16. Heaton, K. W., Manning, A. P., and Hartog, M.: Lack of effect on blood lipid and calcium concentrations of young men on changing from white to wholemeal bread. *Br J Nutr, 35*:55, 1976.

17. Reinhold, J. A., Faradji, B., Abodi, P., and Ismael-Beigi, F.: Decreased absorption of calcium, magnesium, zinc, and phosphorus due to increased fiber and phosphorus consumption as wheat bread. *J Nutr, 106*:493, 1976.

GALLSTONES

Gallbladder stones have been occurring in man and beast for millenia, but only recently has it become clear that the development of cholesterol stones is owing to biochemical abnormalities. Cholesterol stones are the ones most commonly found in our population, and their development requires a bile that is saturated with cholesterol—that substance being present in amounts excessive relative to the concentrations of bile acids and lecithin.[1] Patients with cholesterol gallstones have a decreased body bile-acid pool and an increased rate of secretion of cholesterol into the biliary tree.[2, 3] The bile in such persons is called *lithogenic*. In patients with functioning gallbladders, the gallbladder bile contains more cholesterol and less bile salt than does the common-duct bile.[3] In patients with nonfunctioning gallbladders, the two biles are identical. An interesting finding is that the nonfunctioning gallbladder contains bile that has less cholesterol and more bile acid than the bile in a functioning gallbladder. This general mechanism operates also in obese persons.[4] On the other hand, the high incidence of gallstones in persons who have had ileostomies or ileal resections has not yet been explained.[5]

Lithogenic bile is known to be produced by certain circumstances. One is the use of the diet today recommended by some physicians for lowering the serum cholesterol level. This diet, low in cholesterol and high in polyunsaturated fats, more than doubled the incidence of cholesterol gallstones in one study.[6] The ill-advised use of a markedly distorted diet appears to be responsible for causing gallstones in some people who otherwise would not have them.

Another example of a marked change in regimen causing an increased incidence of gallstones is found in women who take estrogen-containing contraceptive pills. It also is found in postmenopausal women who take estrogen.[7] A study made on normal young women showed that taking oral contraceptive pills caused changes in the constitution of the bile known to favor the formation of cholesterol gallstones.[7] The concentration of cholesterol increased and the bile-acid constitution of the bile changed. Chenodeoxycholic acid decreased, as did lithocholic acid derived from it. Cholic acid increased. The fall in chenodeoxycholic acid content is interesting, since that bile acid has been used to remove gallstones already present.[8, 9] The dose must be at least 10 to 15 mg/kg/per day.[10]

A recently published preliminary report[11] indicates that the ingestion of 57 grams of wheat bran a day lowers the cholesterol saturation of bile, apparently by increasing the formation of chenodeoxycholic acid.

A totally unrelated nutritional phenomenon may be encountered in patients with gallbladder disease. In such patients, ingestion of fat may cause gallbladder contraction unless that organ is too badly damaged. Hence, these patients may vigorously exclude fat from the diet. Vitamin A deficiency may develop in these circumstances. Such patients should take a water-soluble preparation of the vitamin by mouth in a dose of around 3,000 to 5,000 units per day.

REFERENCES

1. Admirand, W. H. and Small, D. M.: The physicochemical basis of cholesterol gallstone formation in man. *J Clin Invest*, 47:1043, 1968.
2. Vlahceric, C. R., Bell, C. C., Jr., Buhac, I.: Diminished bile acid pool size in patients with gallstones. *Gastroenterology*, 59:165, 1970.
3. Antsaklis, G., Lewin, M. R., Sutor, D. J., Cowie, A. G. A., and Clark, C. G.: Gallbladder function, cholesterol stores, and bile composition. *Gut, 16*:937, 1975.
4. Mabee, T. M., Meyer, P., Den Besten, L., and Mason, E. E.: The mechanism of increased gallstone formation in obese human subjects. *Surg, 79*:460, 1976.
5. Hill, G. L., Mair, W. S. J., and Goligher, J. C.: Gallstones after ileostomy and ileal resection. *Gut, 16*:932, 1975.
6. Sturdevant, R. A., Pearce, M. L., and Dayton, S.: Increased prevalence of cholelithrosis in man ingesting a serum-cholesterol lowering diet. *N Engl J Med, 288*:24, 1973.
7. Bennion, L. J., Ginsberg, R. J., Gardnick, M. B., and Bennett, P. H.: Effects of oral contraceptives on the gallbladder bile of normal women. *N Engl J Med, 294*:189, 1974.

8. Bell, G. D., Whitney, H., and Dowling, R. H.: Gallstone dissolution in man using chenodeoxycholic acid. *Lancet*, 2:1213, 1972.
9. Iser, J. H., Dowling, R. H., Mok, H. Y. I., and Bell, G. D.: Chenodeoxycholic acid treatment of gallstones. A follow-up report and analysis of the factors influencing response to therapy. *N Engl J Med*, 293:378, 1975.
10. Thistle, J. L., Hofmann, A. F., Yu, P. Y. S., and Oh, B.: Effect of varying doses of chenodeoxycholic acid on bile lipid and biliary bile acid composition in gallstone patients: a dose-response study. *Dig Dis*, 22:1, 1977.
11. Pomane, E. W., Heaton, K. W., Low-Beer, T. S., and White, C.: Effect of wheat bran on bile salt metabolism and bile composition. *Gut*, 15:824, 1974.

DENTAL CARIES AND GUM DISEASE

T HE MYSTERIES OF dental caries and gum disease have begun to yield to research. The role of nutritional factors in these processes has long been suspected, and at various times such deficiencies as those of calcium or vitamin C have been suggested as causes. However, in uncomplicated cases they do not enter the picture. Epidemiologic studies have long implicated sucrose and perhaps also other carbohydrates as responsible for the formation of dental plaque, the substance responsible for both caries and periodontal disease.[1] Plaque is an adherent gelatinous substance on the teeth. It contains large numbers of bacteria and is made up of bacterial extracellular polysaccharides, leukocytes, salivary glycoproteins, and epithelial remnants.

The metabolism of sucrose by mouth organisms splits that sugar into its component glucose and fructose. The glucose so liberated quickly polymerizes to form a variety of glucans, some of which are of high molecular weight and insoluble; others, smaller and soluble. The former adhere to tooth surfaces and provide an excellent energy source for bacteria. The action of bacteria may also lead to polymerization of the fructose to form so-called levans or fructans. These chemical changes are caused by mouth bacteria, chiefly streptococcus mutants. However, another process appears to be involved in the action of Actinomyces viscosus and related fungi. These organisms adhere to tooth surfaces in the absence of fructose and use other carbohydrates for this purpose. The plaque, whatever its origin, grows down the teeth and along the roots. The bacterial products in it generate an inflammatory reaction which makes the gum pull away, allowing more bacterial penetration.

The gelatinous, adherent carbohydrate polymer stimulates the adhesion and growth of the organisms on the tooth surfaces. The organisms grow anaerobically, and ferment the substrate to lactic and other acids. The plaque has an acid pH and the acid products of fermentation attack the enamel. In addition, the micro-organisms produce a variety of lytic enzymes, toxins, and antigens which are also destructive.

It is evident that the amount of carbohydrate, especially sucrose, ingested must influence the frequency and severity of plaque formation and, hence, of dental caries and gingivitis. It is also apparent that only by assiduous tooth cleaning can the plaque that forms be removed.

The possible role of carbohydrates other than sucrose has recently been denied.[2] In observations made by Hankin et al.[2] on Hawaiian, Japanese, and Caucasian children, the amount of dental caries varied from group to group, but in all of them eating bread, rolls, buns, and breakfast cereal between meals was negatively correlated with the amount of caries, whereas the between-meal eating of candy was positively correlated with dental caries.

The role of minerals in gum disease has also been discussed.[3] There was no convincing effect of dietary calcium, phosphorus, or protein, or of trace metals or vitamins. The same was true of serum levels. No measurement of fluoride or strontium contents (page 82) was made.

Sugar still seems to be the main offender.

REFERENCES

1. Brown, A. T.: The role of dietary carbohydrates in plaque formation and oral disease. *Nutr Rev, 33*:353, 1975.
2. Hankin, J. H., Chung, C. S., and Kan, M. C. W.: *J Dent Res, 52*:1079, 1973.
3. Freedland, J. H., Cousins, R. J., and Schwartz, R.: Relationship of mineral status and intake to periodontal disease. *Am J Clin Nutr, 29*:745, 1976.

OXALATE METABOLISM —
URINARY CALCULI

Oxalate is widely distributed in plants, comprising, in some, as much as 20 percent of the dry weight. Plants contain both insoluble oxalate (chiefly the calcium salt) and soluble oxalate (the sodium and potassium salts). Considerable amounts of oxalate may be taken in cocoa, tea, chocolate, and in vegetables, e.g. rhubarb and spinach. However, only 2 to 5 percent of ingested oxalate is absorbed, and this is excreted in the urine. Increased amounts of oxalate are absorbed from the gut in patients with ileal resections, small bowel disease, and with steatorrhea caused by a variety of intestinal diseases.[1] In the latter cases, the sequestration of calcium by the fat decreases the formation of insoluble calcium oxalate, leaving the oxalate free to be absorbed. The absorption of this oxalate requires that colonic function be normal,[2] for the colon is the site of the absorption of the oxalate. In addition, oxalate is formed in man as an end product of certain metabolic processes. The major part of oxalate in the urine is normally formed endogenously, the principal sources being ascorbate and glyoxylate, the latter derived mainly from glycine. Small amounts come from glycolic acid and from amino acids other than glycine. Hydroxyproline is also a source, ordinarily unimportant, but becoming increasingly significant in persons with high hydroxyproline outputs, i.e. normal children and persons who are making large amounts of collagen. The metabolic pathways responsible for oxalate production in man are described in detail by Hagler and Herman.[3] Hyperoxaluria is produced by vitamin B_6 deficiency, especially in the presence of a high tryptophan intake.[4] Thiamine deficiency may also lead to increased oxalate formation, but this does not seem to be important in man.[5]

Calcium oxalate may be found as crystals in freshly voided urine from normal persons when the urine pH is below 6.2.

However, most of the oxalate is in solution and may be ionized. A few apparently normal persons excrete somewhat increased amounts. Persons with hypercalciuria from one cause or another excrete increased amounts of calcium oxalate in the urine. In them the formation of calcium oxalate stones is part of the disease in which abnormal calciuria occurs.

The fascinating, and to some extent puzzling, details of oxalate metabolism enter directly very little into the substance of clinical thinking; it comes to the fore only in certain poisonings. On the other hand, the metabolism of oxalate is of great concern to clinicians who encounter patients with urinary calculi, even though the metabolic fate of oxalate does not explain the occurrence of stones. This discussion does not refer to the stones that occur in association with infection; these consist mainly of magnesium ammonium phosphate. The stones to be discussed here occur in patients with sterile urine and, at least initially, an anatomically normal unobstructed urinary tract. Such patients are most numerous in the "stone belt" in the mid-Atlantic and southeastern states. In such patients about 70 percent of the stones contain calcium oxalate mainly with lesser amounts of crystalline phosphate.[6] The growth of the crystals that form these stones was studied by Pak and Holt.[7] Over 80 percent of bladder stones in children in endemic areas, e.g. Southeast Asia, have a similar constitution.[8] However, the endemic bladder stone disease of the Far East seems to be so special in its distribution and its clinical characteristics as to make its inclusion in the present discussion unwarranted.[9, 10] It is true that some patients with kidney stones are excreting excessive amounts of calcium in the urine owing to parathyroid disease or bone disease. Others may be putting out increased amounts of uric acid. Some may have disorders that cause increased excretion of hydroxyproline. Some may have unsuspected cadmium intoxication.[11] However, most patients with renal stone disease, in the absence of infection, have no detectable metabolic disorder and, of course, except for the symptoms of the stone itself, no illness of any kind. The urine in such cases must be abnormal in some way. It is interesting that stones are uncommon in women unless a congenital anomaly or an infection is present during the age of ovarian function. During this period of their lives they put out far more citrate in their urine than do men. Citrate keeps calcium in solution.

Some physicians are likely to encounter difficulties in attempting to deal with a disease which cannot be characterized physiologically or biochemically. It is, therefore, interesting to find that an apparently successful nutritional approach to idiopathic renal stone disease is at hand. About fifteen years ago a discovery was made that feeding magnesium oxide depressed renal calculus formation. There are now a number of studies in this area, the most recent of which is by Prien and Gershoff.[12] The patients are given 100 mg of magnesium oxide three times a day plus a trivial supplement (probably unnecessary) of 10 mg of pyridoxine per day. This regimen apparently decreases stone formation by more than 90 percent. An attempt has been made to explain this finding by a study of the urine of stone-formers.[13] The urine of such persons was found to contain statistically smaller amounts of magnesium and statistically larger amounts of calcium and oxalate. These studies, although significant statistically, do not impress one as physiologically significant. Another approach that has been suggested is to reduce the propensity toward stone formation by reducing the urinary output of calcium. This can be accomplished by giving hydrochlorothiazide in doses of 50 mg twice a day.[14]

The mystery of idiopathic renal stone disease has not been solved. However, a nutritional treatment is perhaps at hand, and this may not only benefit the patients but also elucidate the mystery.

REFERENCES

1. Earnest, D. L., Williams, H. E., and Admirand, W. H.: A Physicochemical basis for treatment of enteric hyperoxaluria. *Trans Assoc Am Physicians, 88*:224, 1975.
2. Dobbins, J. W. and Bender, H. J.: Importance of the colon in enteric hyperoxaluria. *N Engl J Med, 296*:290, 1977.
3. Hagler, L. and Herman, R. H.: Oxalate metabolism, I. *Am J Clin Nutr, 26*:758, 1973.
4. Hagler, L. and Herman, R. H.: Oxalate metabolism, II. *Am J Clin Nutr, 26*:882, 1973.
5. Salyer, W. R. and Salyer, D. C.: Thiamine deficiency and oxalosis. *J Clin Pathol, 27*:558, 1974.

6. Prien, E. L. and Prien, E. L., Jr.: Composition and structure of urinary stone. *Am J Med, 45*:654, 1964.
7. Pak, C. Y. C. and Holt, K.: Nucleation and growth of Brushite and calcium oxalate in the urine of stone-formers. *Metabolism, 25*:665, 1976.
8. Gershoff, S. N., Prien, E. L., and Chandrapanond, A.: Urinary stones in Thailand. *J Urol, 90*:285, 1963.
9. Dhanamitta, S., Valyasevi, A., and Van Reen, R.: Studies of bladder stone disease in Thailand. XI. Effect of 4-hydroxy-L-proline and orthophosphate supplementation on crystalluria. *Am J Clin Nutr, 23*:371, 1970.
10. Van Reen, R.: Urinary bladder stone disease. *Proc Ninth Intern Cong Nutrition (Mexico), 1*:259, 1972.
11. Scott, R., Patterson, P. J., Mills, E. A., McKirdy, A., Fell, G. S., Ottoway, J. M., Husaim, F. E. R., Fitzgerald-Finch, O. P., Yates, A. J., Lamont, A., and Roxburgh, S.: Clinical and biochemial abnormalities in coppersmiths exposed to cadmium. *Lancet, 2*:396, 1976.
12. Prien, E. L. and Gershoff, S. F.: Magnesium oxide-pyridoxine therapy for recurrent calcium oxalate calculi. *J Urol, 112*:509, 1974.
13. Hodgkinson, A.: Relations between oxalic acid, calcium, magnesium, and creatinine excretion in male patients with calcium oxalate kidney stones. *Clin Sci Molec Med, 46*:357, 1974.

XANTHOMATOSIS

Xanthomas are well known as cutaneous masses of cells filled with cholesterol-esters. These cutaneous (or, occasionally, ligamentous) nodules or plaques are found in some, evidently a minority, patients with high serum cholesterol levels. On the other hand, many of the patients who exhibit these cutaneous changes have normal serum cholesterol levels. Moreover, in most instances decreasing the cholesterol intake does not decrease the size or number of the xanthomas.

A possible explanation for these inconsistencies has recently been brought forward by recent studies in what seems to be a rare condition. In this disorder, although the xanthomas consist almost entirely of cholesterol-esters, their formation appears to be associated with the absorption of the plant sterol, beta-sitosterol.[1] To what extent this peculiar physiologic disorder participates in the genesis of xanthomas in general is not known. Nevertheless, the fact that a plant sterol can cause deposition of cholesterol-esters in tissues despite normal serum cholesterol levels should not be ignored in view of the current practice of taking increased amounts of vegetable oils in the diet.

REFERENCES

1. Shulman, R. S., Bhattachayya, A. K., Connor, W. E., and Fredrickson, D. S.: β-sitosterolemia and xanthomatosis. N Engl J Med, 294:482, 1976.

INDEX